30

(H)

THE ROAD
TO
SHANGRI-LA

THE ROAD TO SHANGRI-LA

My 60,000 Mile Quest For
The Secrets of Rejuvenation

Ann Beveridge

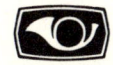

Arlington Books
Clifford Street, Mayfair
London

THE ROAD TO SHANGRI-LA
first published 1979 by
Arlington Books (Publishers) Ltd
3 Clifford Street Mayfair
London W.1.

© *Ann Beveridge 1979*

Set in England by
Inforum Ltd Portsmouth
Printed and bound in England by
Billing & Sons Ltd
Guildford, Worcester and London

British Library Cataloguing in Publication Data
Beveridge, Ann
The road to Shangri-La.
1. Rejuvenation
I. Title
613   QP90
ISBN 0–85140–477–4

CONTENTS

Acknowledgements

My sincere thanks are due to the following:

Professor Dr Ana Aslan, Director General, National Institute of Gerontology and Geriatrics, Romania; Dr Thomas Beck, Sydney, Australia; Dr Dean Burk, (formerly Chief Chemist, Department of Cell Chemistry, National Cancer Institute, Washington; The Cancer Control Society of America; The Center for Life Extension and Control of Ageing, Sacramento, California; Dr Alexander Ciuca, Director, National Institute of Gerontology and Geriatrics, Romania; Dr Alex Comfort, Center for the Study of Democratic Institutions, Santa Barbara, California; Dr W. Donner Denckla, Chief Biochemist, Roche Institute of Molecular Biology, Nutley, N.J.; Professor Yu. A. Dobrovolski, Leningrad; Mr Michael Edgley, Australia; Dafna Edwards, Los Angeles; Dr Caleb E. Finch, Associate Professor, Laboratory of Neurobiology, Andrus Gerontology Center, University of Southern California, Los Angeles; Dr Bernard Grad, McGill University, Montreal, Canada, (for help on his theories of Life Energy); Dr Harold Harper, Los Angeles, (for help in Chelation Therapy and the problems of ageing); Mr Frederick A. Jeffriess, Hyperbaric Systems, Vickers Medical, Basingstoke, England; Dr Ernst T. Krebs, Jnr., The John Beard Memorial Foundation, San Francisco, California; Dr Hans Kugler, American Biochemist, (for help with research on Gerontology); Mr Phillip Lebon, London Plastic Surgeon; Dr Evin Lopreiss, U.S. Navy Research Department, Long Beach, California, (for help on Hyperbaric Medicine); Dr Sigrid Lohmann, Kuratorium Deutsche Altershilfe, Cologne; Mr Andrew R.L.

McNaughton, The McNaughton Foundation, California; News Limited, Australia and *The Sydney Daily Telegraph*; Novosti News Bureau, Moscow; Pakistan International Airlines; Dr Linus Pauling, Director, Institute of Orthomolecular Medicine, Menlo Park, California; Dr Gaston L.S. Pawan, Metabolic Division, Department of Medicine and Institute of Clinical Research, Middlesex Hospital Medical School, London; Mr Vidal Sassoon, Los Angeles; Schwartzhaupt, Cologne; The Rt. Hon. Ian Sinclair, Australia; Mr Roland W. Steinbach, Schwartzhaupt, Cologne; Dr Joachim Stein, Heidelberg, West Germany, Vice-President of the International Society For Research on Cell Therapy; Dr Peter Stephan, Harley Street, London; U.C.L.A. Biomedical Library, California; Dr Fritz Wiedemann, Sanatorium Wiedemann, Bavaria; Mr David Wilkinson, British Airways; Mr D.P.A. (Bill) Wilson, Sydney, Australia; Dr Steven Zax, Hollywood Plastic Surgeon.

I should also like to express my tremendous gratitude to all the scores of other people throughout the world for their patience and help, without which this book would not have been possible. In particular, my parents, for their unfailing encouragement and support.

Foreword

Just how much chance have *you* of hanging onto youth beyond the years nature allocates? Do youth drugs and youth treatments really exist?

Have scientists actually found the panacea, the wonder cure, which would keep us young forever that they have claimed for so long to be on the verge of discovery?

Is longevity, the chance of living healthily to be 120 or 200 or even 1,000 years of age, still an idea that belongs only to the realms of science fiction?

Today – more than at any other time in our history – to stay young, to hang on to our youth longer, to be seen to be youthful has never been more vital.

Women have never before been so terrified of the first sign of wrinkles, sagging figures or greying hair as marriage becomes an increasingly unstable institution and Women's Lib has, as yet, failed to provide a secure alternative, particularly to the mother of a young family.

Men, equally, fear the loss of their boyish looks, middle-aged spread and – even worse – the loss of their sex drive, which in turn means the threat of losing their high powered jobs as well as the girls to younger men.

Every year thousands of men and women criss-cross the world searching for the Fountain of Youth. Millions grasp at any little straw of hope – pills, potions, wrinkle creams – anything that would mean a chance of staying younger for longer.

Many of them claim they do look and feel 15 to 20 years younger than they actually are; others like Marlene Dietrich attribute their youthful glamour to cell therapy. She has made no secret of the fact that every few years she has injections from the cells of unborn lambs. Others report their own methods of achieving glowing, newly youthful complexions, the lessening of wrinkles, a return of a new vitality, sparkling health and often an exciting new sex life.

Where do they go, what treatments are being held out, how many of them work and which are purely the offerings of quacks and charlatans anxious to make a quick buck out of desperate customers who seek youth at any price?

A year ago I quite accidentally lifted the lid off the world of the youth doctors, and found a fantastic multi-billion dollar business operating all over the world. I decided it was time somebody found out the facts, the whole truth about what is going on in the, until now, secret medical world of which few people ever talk and about the youth doctors whose work for the most part has been wrapped in a conspiracy of silence. I set out to unwrap the world of the gerontologist, the scientists of the 21st century who are at this moment solving the secrets of our future and the way we will live it.

We are all poised on the tip of a Brave New World in which the treatments, regarded today as extraordinary and in many cases in the realms of science fiction, will be common-place, every day facts of life for the generations of tomorrow.

You will be amazed at the lengths to which some people are going already to recapture their youth as well as some of the revolutionary new treatments and discoveries being held out to all of us right round the world. You owe it to yourself to know about them.

Ann Beveridge

CHAPTER ONE

Is There A Fountain Of Youth?

"Cicero said over 2,000 years ago: 'The short period of life is yet long enough for living well and honourably . . .'

That was 2,000 years ago. Isn't it time for a new look at our life span and the way we live it?"

Ann Beveridge

Right at the start I'll set the record straight for the disbelievers, the cynics and traditionalists, who prefer to cling to the cobwebbed ideas of the past, and who regard as so much nonsense the theory that there is a Fountain of Youth.

I am no modern day Ponce de Leon, who sought the secret of eternal youth as long ago as the 16th century – and failed. I want to say quite categorically, succinctly and loudly now – after an amazing 60,000 mile journey across the world on the youth treasure trail, talking to scientists, doctors, plastic surgeons, molecular biologists, bio-chemists, physicists, immunologists, endocrinologists, psychiatrists and sociologists, all actively engaged in multi-billion dollar programmes to solve the problems of ageing – there IS a 20th century answer to the Fountain of Youth.

Any one of us can, for a price, tap the secrets that will keep old age at bay, and will also help us to live longer and enable us to look forward to an active, healthy, vital and productive old age. I believe quite firmly, as you'll see from my findings, that we *can* turn back the clock; that we *can* look years younger than our actual age; that it *is* possible to prevent wrinkles, and put the elasticity back into ageing skin, improve failing eyesight and memory retention, restore hair colour, solve the balding problem, put the zest back into a jaded sex life and prevent many of the crippling and slowly degenerative diseases that make ageing such a misery for so many.

All of us are egocentrics. We find ourselves, and everything affecting us personally, of prime fascination, and therefore, it has been quite natural for people down the centuries to be intrigued by the riddle of life and death and in particular their own chances of staying young and cheating old age.

Even more intriguing is the subject of longevity. To contemplate the prospect of eternal life, or at least a much increased life span mellowing into golden, enriched later years of fulfilment both mentally and physically, instead of today's indignities, humiliations and senility which sadly, for most of us, are a feared but almost inevitable accompaniment to ageing.

No wonder then that gerontology – the scientific study of ageing – is the most intriguing, fast moving branch of modern science today. For decades gerontologists have had to work on the very fringe of conventional medicine. For the most part their work has been denounced, and they themselves have been pilloried, shunned or ignored by their more traditional medical colleagues. When their discoveries were taken out and examined, what little progress had been made was identified at once with the less reputable shady practitioners, in-for-a-quick-buck youth doctors, quacks and charlatans of whom there have always been plenty, but who only succeeded in discrediting the whole field and putting research back by decades.

Today, however, the problems of ageing have never been more pressing. As the average life span increases and the world population doubles and quadruples so, too, is the crippling financial burden on government resources being stretched ever more widely to cater for the world's older generations.

In hospitals, old peoples' homes, mental institutions, private clinics and nursing homes, as well as through the constant drain on general medical services, the care of the elderly is becoming not only a key financial problem but also a sociological one.

Unfortunately it is a fact, as statistics show at this moment, that as people become older the incidences of diseases increase, doubling about every 8.5 years. In the USA the health care bill is in excess of $150 billion annually – and the figures are rising steeply all the time.

As a result, in the last few years in order to try and stem the flow, before it soars out of all proportion, many more billions of dollars are being allocated to scientists to enable them to try and solve many of the problems of ageing.

Serious research programmes are being undertaken in most of our major countries to solve officially the questions that have intrigued man for all time; the secrets of longevity, of life and even death itself. What the gerontologists are probing is what causes us to start ageing; can they control it, or even better, reverse it; and is there, in fact, a mechanism within our bodies that decides when we will die?

I will try to outline the answers to many of these questions – in some cases with claims that still seem to belong to the realms of science fiction but which, some of our most eminent scientists tell me, are simply the facts of life of the 21st century.

I don't feel I am in any way being an extremist in suggesting that people now over forty will be the last of the generations who believe it is natural and desirable to grow old gracefully. To let nature take its painful course and to allow ourselves to be "clocked out" somewhere around the biblical three scores years and ten.

From what I've discovered, I believe that future generations will be expected to care for their minds and bodies better; that it will be a responsibility to themselves and their families to keep healthy as long as possible into their advancing years and that youth doctors will be as accepted in our medical society as dentists, opticians or chiropodists are today.

Already we are living in a youth-orientated society without precedent. We are bombarded by advertisers, television, press and retailers to believe that if we aren't youthful we aren't in the race. Yet, there comes the day for all of us when we know we are on the treadmill, when we can no longer deny that our bodies aren't quite as good as they used to be; that we don't feel as fit as we once did; that we are overweight, sagging, flabby and probably showing the signs of the good life.

For a woman there may not even be many wrinkles, just laughter lines and character lines that give a face more interest than the flat artist's canvas it is at eighteen. Yet for her it's the start of facials, night creams and moisturising lotions, of spending more money than she used to on flattering make-ups, cover-up creams, hair tints and anything else the manufacturers proclaim will help keep her eternally twenty-seven.

For a man it usually means a half-hearted switch to low calorie beer, the start of morning exercises or jogging, a subscription to a health club, or almost certainly, a new found interest in his cholesterol levels.

To most people it's an inner, nagging worry they scarcely admit to themselves. But it's there. What more can I do? they ask themselves. How can I ask my friends without appearing silly, vain, or, at the worst, neurotic – "How do I STOP my age from showing?"

For a woman the start of the menopause, sagging breasts, and a wrinkled, no longer sexually attractive body, or, for a man baldness and perhaps the loss of his sex drive are indeed real fears which, for most people in the past have remained unsaid. It's too personal, too shameful. *That is old fashioned thinking.* It is important to realise that if you are on the youth trail, that if you want to get in on whatever there is being offered, you're not a freak. Seeking out a youth doctor is not a guilty secret you have to hide and certainly you're not vain.

I like top Hollywood plastic surgeon, Steven Zax's view of our desire to improve the way we look: "It's most certainly not vanity," he says sharply, "it's a question of pride. Pride in the way you present yourself to the world."

And what could be wrong with that!

Chapter Two

My Meeting With My First Youth Doctor

"Experimental gerontology may well prove the medical growth stock of the next decade . . ."
Dr Alex Comfort, In "The Mechanisms of Ageing and Development"

I knew nothing of the incredible world of the youth doctors a few years ago. I'd heard, of course, vague mutterings – from my mother in England about monkey glands way back in my childhood, and there was a model I knew in London who nearly died after taking dehydrated tapeworms in order to slim. But for the most part youth "cures" and quackery were, in my mind, synonymous.

I had no idea of the extent of the fantastic hush-hush, multibillion dollar youth supermarket to which increasing thousands of ordinary people are flocking each year, hoping to buy back their youth by the dollar or the pound.

My meeting with my very first youth doctor happened in Australia in July, 1975. As on all the momentous occasions which turn our thinking upside down, I was totally unprepared for the flood gates of curiosity our meeting was to open for me. I was working as Women's Editor of *The Sydney Daily Telegraph* when a friend rang to invite me for lunch at the Hilton Hotel. There was a man, he said, whom he thought I would be fascinated to meet.

We were to gather beforehand in the foyer of a city medical centre but as I glided smoothly upwards in the elevator I had no way of knowing that I was about to risk my security, my career, and what laughingly passed as my bank balance and spin off in a time capsule into a world which revolves around knocking years off people's lives.

The neat stainless steel plate outside the double glass doors gave no clue. It read simply "Obesity and Gerontology Centre". "Uh huh," I groaned to myself. "They're after publicity for another slimming treatment." The word *gerontology* was new to me, but I had no time to worry about it as I glimpsed the little group of people quietly waiting in one corner. The man who was introduced to me as Dr Thomas Beck was slight, dapper and immaculately dressed. He was wearing a French cut dark suit, tinted gold-rimmed glasses and a quiet gentle smile. He was smoking a pipe and looked much younger than his forty-eight years.

When I look back on it, all the people who joined us round the lunch table that day looked younger than they in fact were but I didn't attach any particular significance to it then. Between pleasantries and politics they were all talking about something called HCG and a Russian Vitamin – B15. It all sounded terribly technical and I couldn't contribute much to the conversation.

But I did take a lot of notice of what the Czech-born, softly accented Dr Beck was telling me. Did I know, he said, that the Russians had discovered that they could extend the human life span over several hundred years? Beat that for a conversation starter!

I didn't know it then but I was hooked – hook, line and sinker on the youth kick. I wanted to know more and I was pretty sure that most other thinking men and women over the age of twenty-five and certainly over thirty-five would want to know more too.

Dr Beck was, at that time, running a chain of very successful slimming and revitalisation clinics in Australia and, when I wrote about them in a series of newspaper articles a short time later, women in their hundreds queued to get through his door for treatment. No, I wasn't wrong. People everywhere were wanting the answers to the new big super question of today. Is there something in the youth market for them?

Within months I was flying the world with a full appointment book, heading to see top doctors, scientists and gerontologists, hoping one would lead me to another on a trail that literally took me to the four corners of the globe.

My aim: to find out *everything* there is to know about the youth treatments available and the revolutionary work scientists are doing to increase our chances of rejuvenation and longevity in the future.

It was a mind–bending journey. My route took me from the film star homes of Hollywood to the dank corridors of Europe's oldest hospital deep in Soviet Russia; from a tropical holiday island paradise off the North-East coast of Australia to the seedy, dusty backstreets of a Mexican border town; from suburban New Jersey to the Far East and Japan, as well as to some of the best equipped rejuvenation clinics in the world in Germany, Romania, London and South America to which patients pour annually in their thousands seeking the *Jungkur* "Cure".

CHAPTER THREE

The Youth Supermarket:
The Film Stars Who Go There

"While getting old is inevitable, it can be slowed."
Dr E. Cheraskin and Dr W M Ringsdorf, Jnr.

The further I travelled the more astonished I became by the vast numbers of people who, each year, circle the world looking for ways of keeping young, usually under cover of taking a package holiday.

They are not all millionaires and film stars, far from it, although admittedly, the rich and famous managed to keep the most successful youth doctors of all expensively and exclusively to themselves until the last decade.

Today the youth market is aimed at men and women from all walks of life, who want to present themselves to the world in as good, youthful and healthy a state as possible for as long as possible. The youth trail is their only hope and it can be a confusing and unnerving one for the uninitiated.

Certainly it involved me in some hair-raising excapades. Like the time I became unwittingly involved in the cancer drug-smuggling ring between Mexico and the U.S.A.; like the three days I spent alone in Bucharest waiting to see Romania's famous Professor Dr Ana Aslan and was slipped a "Mickey Finn" in a Bucharest night club.

Often I wondered what in heavens name I was doing, after driving three hundred miles by road and then standing for half an hour in front of a plastic statue of a tennis player in Tijuana's sleazy main street waiting for a mysterious Mexican youth doctor to pick me up. The only thing I knew about him was his name and phone number.

On another occasion a top London plastic surgeon bawled me out and reduced me to tears, jetlagged and fatigued as I was after weeks of travelling. Then he changed his mind after I wrote to him from Germany and spent three hard working evenings telling me all the secrets of his surgeon's knife. You can read the results – in our blow-by-blow interview: what exactly you can expect from a face lift, nose bobbing, eye debagging, tummy and bottom lifting and enlarging or reshaping of the breasts. He told me, too, about some of his most incredible patients, about penis implants, which can revitalize a man's sex life and his revolutionary way of curing baldness.

I spent long hours, too, with Hollywood's priciest plastic surgeon, the glamorous Steven Zax – the man whose hands shape the faces and figures of the stars. We talked about his work, his super plush surgery with its secret side door for the stars and a third door for his clientele when the press are watching the second.

At the same time I visited the world's top hairdresser, the eternally youthful looking Vidal Sassoon who, with his actress wife, Beverly, knows more than most about what the Hollywood Beautiful People are doing behind the scenes to retain their looks.

In some cases I tracked down the story of an individual treatment from one side of the world to the other, to check out its history and effects. Treatments like the world famous cell therapy, intra-muscular injections using cells from unborn lambs discovered by the internationally-known Professor Paul Niehans. I traced its origins to the luxurious and exclusive La Prairie clinic in Switzerland to which the rich and famous, potentates and film stars have gone in their scores since the nineteen-thirties to keep themselves eternally young.

I travelled to Berlin to see one of the leading exponents of the treatment, Dr Joachim Stein, and followed him back to Heidelberg to see the fascinating laboratories where the sheep are slaughtered and the lyophilised, or freeze dried, cells go out to thousands of doctors all over the world. There are over 6000 general practitioners using cell therapy in West Germany today alone.

I went to a remote island in the South Pacific where I discovered the secrets of cell therapy first-hand in a tropical holiday paradise where the famous go in disguise. I met, too, many of the patients who fly each year to Dr Ana Aslan's famous Fountain of Youth in Romania. She proclaims the merits of her Procaine based youth jabs, Gerovital, still the subject of world-wide medical controversy. Does it work?

Thousands of ordinary people, who buy the treatment in pill form over their chemist's counter in Europe and elsewhere, believe it does, and today the Aslan formula is being administered to 200,000 Romanian factory workers in a giant experiment to examine their work capacity, efficiency and vitality compared with men and women not on the jabs.

I flew on to see one of the world's most luxurious millionaire-style clinics run by Dr Fritz Wiedemann in the beautiful depths of the Bavarian Alps. American tourists go there annually by the jumbo jet-load to undergo his ten day multi-treatment cure. It is based mainly on Bogomoletz serum – rejuvenating injections developed by the Russians to keep Stalin alive. It is an amazing picture book scene of flowers and old world chalets where, in an almost Peter Pan atmosphere of timelessness, patients walk in the sunshine or relax beside a film star swimming pool under brightly coloured umbrellas, waiting for their "cure" to work.

There were some pretty off-beat ideas, too, which I shall be telling you about, like fertilised chicken eggs in the Bahamas, which patients swallow whole; and fertilised turtle eggs in the South Pacific, said to prolong youth. There was Chile's famous FGF-60 treatment used by many famous stars, Mexico's blood washing and I mustn't forget the French doctor in New Caledonia who claims he can inject cells direct into facial wrinkles and make them vanish for up to a year!

Then there are the many diet clinics using HCG, hormone extracts from the urine of pregnant women, said to cause fast weight loss from all the difficult places normal diets don't reach – the inner thighs, under-arms, bottom and hips.

I looked into many important theories on nutrition, particularly in relation to diseases like cancer and arthritis; into acupuncture, into chelation therapy, sea water and mud therapies, bio-feedback and body servicing and RNA and DNA revitalisation treatments.

Some of the most fascinating and revolutionary new treatments just filtering out now are being achieved with the use of Hyperbaric Chambers, HBO, using one hundred per cent pure oxygen given to patients in a special unit, like an iron lung, enabling it to be administered at below sea level pressures. It was developed originally by the U.S. Navy for use in underwater medicine to treat divers with bad cases of the 'bends'. Now some side effects are being shown to have amazing possibilities for revitalisation and executive brush-ups curing baldness, improving memory retention, restoring hair colour and skin tone and dramatically boosting the libido.

The names of the famous who are said to have benefited from some of these youth treatments read like an international *Who's Who*. Most of them have been to either cell therapy clinics in Europe or to undergo the Aslan treatment.

Top people like the late President Kennedy, the Shah of Iran, Marlene Dietrich, the Duchess of Windsor, the Emperor of Japan, Picasso, Gloria Swanson, Elizabeth Taylor, Cary Grant, Frank Sinatra, Kirk Douglas, the late President Kruschev, Sir Winston Churchill, the late President Peron of Argentina and Pope Pius XII are all said to have had youth treatments – and it has never been denied.

Many of today's leading Hollywood film stars, pop stars and television personalities round the world are all into the youth kick wherever and whenever they can get it, although few will admit it even when confronted with "I saw you there" evidence. Still, that's all part of the youth game, and why not?

Now the youth supermarket is open to anyone who saves up the money to go and shop there, but the question is where to go; what clinics are reputable, which treatments really work, which are the right treatments for you personally and your problems; and, most important of all, who are the cheats and get-rich-quick fakes ripping off their gullible patients with quack or quasi remedies.

I can tell you. After extensive and long research into *every* aspect of the treatments, I will describe to you how the theories, the doctors and their results came over to me as a layperson. No doctor in the world is going to stick his neck out and pass comment at risk of his career. As an observer, I can only tell you that I have reported as accurately as is humanly possible.

I'm laying all the evidence before you. After reading my findings your view is up to you . . . but perhaps you'll have a newly enlightened approach to yourself, your body and the way you'll cope with your own advancing years.

CHAPTER FOUR

What Chance Has Any One Of Us Of Reaching The 22nd Century?

"If we control ageing – for example, maintain indefinitely the physiology of a 15-year-old – the average life span would be in excess of 25,000 years."
Bernard Strehler, PhD., University of Southern California

Youth is a curious phenomenon. While we have it we tend to imagine we are physically immortal; that in some mysterious way life, for us, will go on for ever. That, like Peter Pan, we will remain eternally young.

Certainly, all of us in our early years grew impatient with being ignored or disregarded because our elders saw us as too young and inexperienced to be taken seriously. We wished away those precious birthdays, so eager were we for them to listen to what we had to say. But beyond that, in the time capsule of the young mind, the passing of the weeks and years is of no serious consequences. After all, there's a whole life-time ahead to set the world to rights.

But what that life-time means in terms of hours, minutes and seconds has a significance only in the slow frustration of having to wait for something we want like a special treat, a new bicycle, that first pair of long leg trousers or, for a girl, high heeled shoes, and the arrival of Christmas with all its magical surprises. All of us can recall, too, the agony of watching the second hand tick away the time on the school clock during that important examination when all the facts we'd swotted up the night before seemed mysteriously to have vanished.

In our twenties it is much the same. There is always tomorrow to fulfil those vital ambitions and dreams. I can recall that my only pressing aim was to climb fast to the top of the tree so that I could retire at a decrepit thirty which seemed to me, then, to be the ultimate in old age. Except that I didn't picture myself as aged, but living out the rest of my life in a sort of Lotus Eaters never-never-land somewhere in the sun.

In terms of passing years, in relation to the human life span, I'm convinced it is not until a man or woman reaches their early thirties that time has any real meaning. It is not until the spectre of approaching middle-age rears its ugly, unwanted head, when we suddenly realise there is so much to do, see, achieve and experience in much too short a time and that we really are growing older; because when we consider the maximum life span and delete the years of youth and old age, what is left as a fully functional life span in the middle is very short indeed.

But until this point in our awareness is realised, age and ageing is probably best summed up by the definition that anyone ten years older than ourselves – is old!

Scientists tell us that in the development of the human organism we go through two specific and distinct stages: the ascending period up to when we are 30 to 35, a period of growth and development without ageing; and the following descending period from when we begin a steady, predictable decline, slowly but surely degenerating into progressive stages of senescence, disease and eventual death, as part of our natural evolution. Unfortunately, this is natural, but whether it is healthy and necessary is another matter.

After 30, it is an accepted fact that there is a logarithmic increase in the likelihood of dying. Our chances of dying double about every eight years, no matter how fit and healthy we may try to keep ourselves. It would seem therefore, that in some strange, maybe only subconscious way, that our interest in ourselves, our bodies and how long we may live does coincide with the start of our descending period or more specifically, the beginning of the end.

In the past, I suppose, to pause to consider our life expectancy was a bit of a morbid waste of time. After all – what on earth was the point? But that was before scientists got down to digging up some of the startling new facts with which they are now confronting us and each other. Many of them now believe that science could be on the verge of a revolutionary, radical discovery in unravelling the secrets behind why we age, why we die and ultimately how to reverse the whole process and keep us eternally young.

So what, then, are the chances of any one of US living to see the 22nd century? Is it possible that before too long man will expect to reach not only the 100 mark with ease, but 200, 500 or 1000 years of age? And that doesn't mean a life time of being old but an active youthful life span without any of the crippling, miserable diseases of ageing known to man today.

Preposterous though these ideas may seem, don't scoff at them too soon. Remember, it's not so very long ago that we were laughing at the idea of man ever flying to the moon . . .

At least one brilliant young American scientist believes that some of us almost certainly could be around to see the year 3,001 – because he claims he has already found the secret of eternal life. Dr Donner Denckla is chief Biochemist at the world famous Roche Institute of Molecular Biology in Nutley, New Jersey in America. Heading a research programme into the problems of ageing, he says he has discovered a new hormone secreted in the vital pituitary gland at the base of the skull which he claims holds the whole secret of life and death.

Dr Denckla, a tall, intense fast-talking American is a family man with his feet very firmly on 20th century *terra firma*, despite his mind-boggling claims. He is one of a large school of international scientists who have believed for some time in the theory that each individual life span is programmed by a "time clock of ageing" in the brain which, when triggered, ensures we die on or around our allotted time. Dr Denckla says the previously unknown hormone he has pinpointed – he calls it, for want of a better name, a decreasing oxygen consumption hormone – cloaks at a certain point the rest of the bodily systems that are the key for survival. This means we then clock out or die. Death therefore, for most of us is a precisely timed event.

At present Dr Denckla is working on taking out the pituitary gland, isolating the hormone and either leaving out or reprogramming it. If he can do it, technically man could live for ever. Is it possible?

According to the biochemist, who is regarded by colleagues as one of the most inventive brains in the business it is already theoretically done. It's just a case, he says, of man hours, technical assistance and patience. But Dr Denckla has no doubt that it will be achieved and in a very short time.

In addition, Dr Denckla threw in, as if for good measure, a further startling discovery. That he had also found the method of reversing ageing in rats and mice. He has brought old rats of the equivalent of 60 human years back to a youthful 20 again. It's mind-bending stuff, isn't it? It has such far reaching sociological, emotional, ecological and economic implications that it would challenge even our greatest thinkers. For a start we would face a population problem of unparalleled proportions. It would create the greatest upheaval mankind has ever had to consider.

However, since this book is all about what you and I can do now, this instant, to make us look and feel better I'll leave the details of that one for later on. As it is unlikely that such a world shattering discovery would be released by world health authorities at all – and certainly not in the immediate future – let's concentrate instead on today. Let's take a look on a more practical level at our chances of longer life.

Statistics show quite clearly that the average life span for people throughout the world has increased significantly during the 20th century. This is due mainly to environmental controls and the great advances in our knowledge of hygiene, nutrition and general health care. At the moment, however, the probability of most of us ever achieving even that human milestone, the 100 mark, is unlikely unless your parents or grandparents lived well into their nineties.

Most doctors agree under present medical rules that that is a pretty accurate yardstick whereby to measure your own life span.

Russian scientists are among many who are loud in their assertions that the specific genetic code of longevity is hereditary. Headed by one of the world's best known gerontologists, Professor Dmitri Chebotarev, Director of the Russian Institute of Gerontology in Kiev, they believe that the genes actually determine the entire life cycle of each human being; that we are genetically programmed by some sort of built-in pacemaker.

In particular, they determine at what age the descending or degenerative cycle will start in each person, normally somewhere after 25 but usually between 30 and 35. For example, in mongoloids who are born with 47 chromosomes per cell instead of 46, as in the normal adult human being, and who manufacture a thousand different enzymes in 50% greater quantity than normal persons, the ageing process is observed to be much more rapid than in other people.

Chebotarev says that centenarians are the best example of adaptation to ageing. In the main centenarians are the product of parents who themselves lived to 100 or more, and they all exhibit such a smooth development of degeneration that when it does occur there is no sudden wearing out of vital organs and functions such as the cardio-vascular or nervous systems. As a result, the individual generally remains biologically younger than his or her chronological or actual years.

In Russia today, for example, there are around 19,000 people who are over 100 years old, many of them living in the Caucasus region of the U.S.S.R., famous for its large numbers of long lived, active and independent inhabitants. In some parts of the region approximately 100 out of every 100,000 people are over a 100 years old. Presently, the average life span in the U.S.S.R. as a whole is 70 to 72 compared with only 32 as short a time as 50 years ago.

In the rest of the major industrial countries of the world also, instead of the traditional three score years and ten, people are now regularly living to a riper old age. It's commonplace as we all know to find people in their eighties and nineties.

However, many more doctors and scientists today are now stating their belief that 120 or 200 years of age is a more realistic natural life expectation for which many more of us could reach out and achieve. It's a pretty revolutionary concept and an idea which, I imagine, fills most people with horror.

I'm pretty confident that if I asked any single person in the street today if they would like an opportunity to live to 120, 200 or more, they would cringe and almost certainly reject the idea. The reason for this is that they imagine their old age at the normal 70 mark and believe they would remain in retirement and misery for almost a century. A fate, indeed, worse than death!

But that is not what scientists have in mind at all. They are predicting that many more of us will look forward to much healthier, happier, active, advanced years in which most of the diseases associated with ageing will be non existent; in which all our faculties will remain in full working order and in which mentally, physically, sexually and emotionally we can remain as valued and respected, useful members of the community.

The Center for Life Extension and The Control of Ageing in Sacramento, California, says specifically that current advances in science now make it possible to regard ageing as a disease, subject to treatment and eventual cure. They say it is only a matter of time before scientists unravel the problems of mechanisms of ageing. In the meantime it is likely that extension of human longevity will be achieved by a number of gradual steps because of the many contributory factors involved in the ageing process.

Once ageing is controlled then our susceptibility to disease, chronic disorders and accidents will be greatly reduced and the life span substantially increased. This is why scientists all over the world in most major industrial countries are currently involved in top priority multi-billion dollar research programmes into the problems of ageing.

Each decade, as the world population increases by still more alarming proportions, so, too, do the medical bills. In the U.S., for example, the Government spend around $150 billion a year on health care compared with only $12 billion 10 years ago. No wonder, then, that in 1974 they produced a new *Research into Ageing Act* which resulted in the creation of a new National Institute on Ageing. It has as its nerve centre the flourishing Gerontology Research Center in Baltimore where they carry out a vigorous research programme on the biochemistry, cytology, physiology and psychology of the ageing process. At the moment $15 million a year is being spent on research and much more is needed.

And throughout the rest of the world in Britain, Europe, Australia, Japan and the communist countries in the Eastern European bloc, similar researches are being carried out. Their work falls

into three main categories:
1. Ways to slow the ageing process. In lay terms that is currently the most useful for you and me as it means methods of rejuvenation or, as doctors prefer to call it, revitalisation or regeneration which can knock up to 20 years off our chronological or actual age.
2. Ways to curb, combat and prevent the main diseases of ageing, and main cause of death today: cancer and heart and circulatory diseases.
3. What causes death, in the hope that by understanding its mechanisms they can defuse or reprogramme it to extend to the life span of our choice and ultimate reversal of the ageing process.

They are all aiming to produce a new society in which age is no longer a problem; where living life to the full means just that.

All of us can point to somebody who is 35 and behaves like a person of 55, or conversely to someone who is chronologically 70 and looks 40. Equally, if there is anyone in the world who is 80 and behaves like someone of 50 then it proves one important point: it is possible to be chronologically 80 and be physiologically 50. Which gives all of us the hope that we need.

Nobel Prize winner, Dr Linus Pauling, an American expert on nutrition and Director of the Institute of Orthomolecular Medicine in Menlo Park, California, and himself a septuagenarian, says he believes that most people can achieve an increase of an average of as much as 20 years in the length of the period of well-being and of life.

Correct nutrition and diet can in many cases reduce and retard the diseases of ageing and certainly increase longevity. For example, there is certainly some evidence to show that calorific reduction in several lower animal species will prolong life and that an adequate level of vitamins C and E will slow if not reverse the ageing process.

An eminent nutrition expert, Dr Roger J. Williams, Professor of Biochemistry at the University of Texas, says that many of the diseases and bodily failings caused by ageing could be slowed down if not entirely avoided by proper nutrition. Pointing in particular to the most common characteristics of ageing, impaired vision, hearing, memory, strength and endurance, insomnia, loss of libido, lack of interest in food, aches, pains, increased tendencies towards problems like constipation, diabetes, arteriosclerosis, arthritis and senility etc, he said:

"I want to call attention to the fact that every one of these signs of old age is probably connected with failure of the cells and tissues somewhere in the body to perform their functions properly and also that every one of these failures is related to cell and tissue nutrition . . . We can state with assurance that the longer cells are furnished with the necessities of life including good nutrition the longer they will continue to remain in good working order."

Dr Pauling is a much quoted advocate of the value of the use of vitamins C and E in cutting down the incidence of disease and chance of death at a given age, by one half. We'll look into this in depth in a later chapter on the importance of nutrition, diet and slimming.

However, in a fascinating survey on ageing and death Dr Pauling observes that no matter how careful we are there is no guarantee that we won't die in a car or commercial plane crash or from a disease for which no cure is known.

He makes some interesting comparisons, too, which are surprising, on life expectancy statistics in various countries: despite its highly publicised image as the healthiest, happiest and most affluent society in the world the United States does not have a greater life expectancy rate. Other countries like England, Norway, Denmark, Sweden and Holland exceed the average American life span by 3 to 4 years. The U.S., in fact, holds the record for the lowest life expectancy in one area: for the Papagos Indians in Arizona, it is only 17 years.

Cancer is not, as one might expect, the main killer. In the U.S., for example, it causes only about 20% of deaths. Cigarette smoking, however, accounts for a decrease of four years in the life span of the average American. Dr Pauling says that to eliminate cigarette smoking would, in fact, increase the health and longevity of Americans by 50% more, than to obtain complete control of cancer. If both cancer and cigarettes were controlled the life expectation of Americans would be increased by 6.8 years.

However, none of the advice and revitalising techniques detailed in the following chapters will be of much use to you if you snuff it as a result of air travel, a car accident and/or cigarette smoking.

I throw in the following logistics from Dr Pauling because I find them one of the most amusing pieces of deduction I have come across:

"How much chance of decreasing your life expectancy do you take when you decide to make a trip by air? A jet plane now travels about 500 miles per hour. The number of deaths in commercial air travel leads at once to the conclusion that the decrease in life expectancy resulting from the decision to make the trip by air is about 1 hour per hour travelled. On the other hand, smoking a pack of cigarettes per day for 40 years decreases life expectancy by 8 years; smoking one pack accordingly decreases life expectancy by one fifth of a day, 4.8 hours – which is 14.4 minutes per cigarette smoked. I have measured the length of time required to smoke a cigarette, and have found it to be about 4.8 minutes. Accordingly, the process of smoking a cigarette involves a decrease in life expectancy for the smoker which is three times the time required to smoke the cigarette: smoking cigarettes is three times as dangerous as travelling in a jet plane. Travelling in a jet plane while smoking a cigarette is four times as dangerous as travelling in a jet plane and not smoking. If you fly in an airplane and don't smoke cigarettes you are three times as safe as if you stay at home and smoke cigarettes, or four times as safe as if you fly in an airplane and also smoke. I think that this is a very interesting comparison which all people – all young people especially – ought to know: for whatever length of time they devote to smoking cigarettes they are losing three times that much time from their life."

CHAPTER FIVE

What The Russians Are Doing
To Preserve Youth And Prolong Life

"The source of youth is inside each of us, but not all of us know how to use
it . . ."

Khfaf Lasuria, Age 138, Abkhazia, U.S.S.R.

Whenever we speak of longevity most of us think instantly of the
old men of the Caucasus regions of Russia, the world's epi-centre
of longevity. The long lived people throughout the villages in the
foothills of the Caucasus Mountains have a record of riding, shoot-
ing, hard-living and loving oldsters which makes the rest of us
appear to be made of far more fragile stuff.

There are, according to Soviet statistics, more than 297,000
people of ninety years or older in the Soviet Union today. The
majority live in the Caucasian region or, more precisely, the
Nagorny Karabakh region where approximately 100 out of every
100,000 are over a century old.

Typical would be Mikha Jobua, of the Abkhazian village of
Chlou who at 126 years old says he has no idea of the secret of his
long life but his mother lived to 101, his father saw 140 while his
great-uncle must have been all of 200. Mikha still talks with ease
and perfect memory of the Russo-Turkish War of 1877-78, when
he was a young cavalry man of nearly 30, and of the heavy snows of
1911.

Like all his compatriots in the region, Mikha has been riding
since his childhood and if you doubt that it is possible to reach a
healthy, active and joyful old age you should meet some of the
amazing old men of Abkhazia to discover what living life to the full
really means.

It's hardly surprising that the life style of the Caucasus has long been the target of scientists probing the reasons behind their astounding longevity. Naturally, there are many accusations that the old men of the mountains are not averse to subtracting a few years from their birth certificates or adding a few years on to their century mark. Nonetheless it is certainly indisputable that many of the people in this remote and historically indomitable region of Russia really have reached incredible ages of well over 140 and 150.

What is he like, this typical rugged Abkhazian male who considers it normal to go courting at 100 and thinks nothing of marrying for the second or third time at around the 120 mark? He is usually a blue-eyed, proud and handsome man with silver hair – it doesn't turn grey until he is around 70 – broad shoulders and narrow waistline.

He has strong teeth still in excellent condition – he rinses his mouth with water after every meal – and he is still as at home in the saddle as he was as a boy. He will spend his working day sometimes putting in three to four hours a day – even when over 100 – in the typical working pursuits of the area, picking tea on a collective farm, tending sheep in the high mountains and still perhaps joining in two or three week hunts for bear, wild boar or mountain goat.

Even when an aged Abkhazian stops work on the collective farm his work rhythm continues; there is always something to do around the house, mowing or gathering hay, digging the orchard, threading tobacco leaves or driving cattle to the higher pastures. Persuading an oldster to retire is almost an impossibility in the area.

As has often been said, an Abkhazian views work as naturally as life itself. He doesn't have to work, pensions are supplied to satisfy all his needs. But the men of the region never feel a burden to their family or the community. The depressions so common in age are to them unknown and they radiate tranquility. They are respected members of the village Council of Elders and their word is law to all those who are younger than they.

An ordinary family unit in Caucasia would number around five children and twenty grandchildren.

The Caucasian diet provides, if you will forgive the pun, food for thought when considering their longevity. Fat men are unheard of in the region. The calorific value of their diet is slightly less than that in other parts of the Soviet Union. Caucasians eat the equivalent of 1700–1900 calories a day while the average Soviet would eat 2000–2200 – notably less than most of their counterparts in the West, you will notice, where under 2000 calories today is regarded as "diet" proportions.

Soviet scientists point out that Caucasians have by intuition arrived at the dietary proportions recommended to all elderly people by physicians: a reduction in calories by approximately 30%. This is achieved by maintaining the same amounts of proteins and cutting down on carbohydrates and animal fats.

A typical Caucasian diet is high in vitamin content, and fresh vegetables and fruit are eaten all the year round. Meat – beef, goat's flesh and chicken – is eaten in moderation, usually broiled and served no more than once or twice a week. Soups, broths, bouillon, which doctors say excite the nervous system, are not eaten at all. A normal dinner would always include tomatoes, cucumbers, all kinds of edible herbs, spring onions and garlic. There are always abundant fruits on the table – apples, persimmons, pomegranates and grapes and the juice of the pomegranate, rich in vitamin C, is used to season many of their dishes.

Caucasian food on the whole is spicy by European standards but local inhabitants consume as a balance great quantities of bland matsoni, like yoghurt and buttermilk, which they drink instead of water, claiming it to be a better thirst quencher.

Two interesting additions to the Caucasian diet are walnuts, which are their major fat ingredient (containing up to 70% fats) and honey, which almost completely replaces sugar in the Abkhazian diet.

Dry red wine with a low alcohol content is the staple drink as locals take neither coffee nor tea. They enjoy wine with breakfast, dinner and supper although many centenarians also drink a couple of ounces of home made vodka twice a day, guaranteed to put hairs on the puniest chest.

According to Professor Dmitri Chebotarev, head of the Russian Institute of Gerontology in Kiev, capital of the Ukraine, the

Caucasians illustrate perfectly the four cornerstones of longevity. There are no miracles, he says, but the main factors are certain:
1. Hereditary, a genetic factor.
2. Work of long standing that gives satisfaction.
3. Diet, typical of a given geographical zone.
4. A stable mode and rhythm of life worked out in the course of a person's life.

One of the specialists who have been observing the Caucasian life style is Professor Mamed Ibragimov, Director of the Advanced Training Institute for Doctors in Azerbaijan. He considers that premature impotence is one of the main causes of early ageing, a problem which does not exist in the Caucasian region. It is thought that the problem may be accounted for by their diet of walnuts and honey. However, Caucasians marry late, usually not until thirty to thirty-five but their marriages are usually happy and lasting. Oldsters who lose their partners usually marry again and it is rare to find a Caucasian bachelor!

Russian scientists, perhaps not surprisingly, have long been among the world's foremost in the fight against age and ageing. Some of the most famous as well as most criticised rejuvenators have been Russian, dating back to the last century. In European Communist countries as a whole, it is a fair generalisation to say that rejuvenation and the chances of longevity are not regarded with the same suspicion as in the rest of the medical world, but more as commonplace facts of life.

I went to Russia to try and find out some of these facts for myself. Comparatively few papers on their findings have been published to the medical world, and Western scientists I talked to, who have attended gerontology conferences in the U.S.S.R., say they are not convinced their Russian counterparts have been frank or allowed to be honest in their discussions.

Is it true, I wanted to know, that the Russians have already discovered how to extend the life span by several hundred years? Many scientists believe that it is extremely likely. Led by Chebotarev, the Russian researchers today are all focused on solving the mysteries of the genetic code which determines longevity or the number of years each one of us individually will live. If the specific hereditary gene could be reprogrammed then, of course, the life span could be extended indefinitely. But then, like most things Russian, their research into gerontology tends to come under the heading of military secrets.

The Russian in the street, however, is already benefiting from much of the research. Benefits like Vitamin B15, a therapy which can be given in pill or injection form and which, patients claim, makes them look a fantastic ten to fifteen years younger, is commonly available in the U.S.S.R. as in numerous other countries, as are Vitamins Decamevit, also recommended in Russia for the middle-aged.

So, too, are hormone therapies and tissue therapy, similar to cell therapy, in which an extract of placenta produces a favourable stimulating influence on all the body functions. This, too, is administered by intramuscular injection.

Bogomoletz serum, which was developed by the Russian scientist of that name and which is obtained from the tissues of the brain, placenta and heart of young car accident victims, which in turn is injected into rabbits to obtain the serum, is also said to be beneficial in rejuvenation. This is widely available at European clinics and later I'll describe in detail its use at the millionaire Wiedemann Clinic in Bavaria, where thousands of tourists enjoy its benefits each year.

CHAPTER SIX

My Quest For Youth Inside Russia

"It is not obligatory that everyone has to get sick but everyone has to get old."

Professor Ilyia Michnikov

My journey on the Soviet youth trail was, like all things Russian, at one and the same time frustrating and fascinating.

Arriving in Moscow Airport on a flight from Bucharest, after weeks of wangling and waiting in Consulates, worrying over visas and sending frantic unanswered messages through Departments of Foreign Affairs, I wondered if anyone would know or care about the woman journalist on a youth kick. I needn't have worried.

"Miss B-e-v-e-r-i-d-g-e," came the dismembered voice over the Moscow Airport tannoy.

Me?

A fat, blonde lady gesticulated widely at the passport control counter and a young, bespectacled man, who looked just like a journalist anywhere in the world, told me he was Sergei Buranov of the Novosti News Agency. Between them they helped me fill in a declaration form in Russian and catapulted me off with a mad driver heading for a domestic airport and Leningrad.

The fact that I had an appointment in Kiev seemed to cut no ice at all. At the little airport somewhere in out of town Moscow I was disgorged on the sidewalk and abandoned.

Wandering into the little building filled with local peasants, soldiers and sailors and not one single foreigner in sight I tried to decipher the Russian signs.

Leningrad?

I heard a sailor say something that sounded vaguely like it and joined the half-hour long queue. When I reached the desk a million curious stares later, the clerk took one look at my British passport, had a noisy fit and picking up my baggage, yelling volubly in Russian – ran!

I ran after him round the buildings, down the garden and into a large green Intourist hall – where it seemed I should have been in the first place.

A large, butch-looking lady in a blue uniform told me I had missed my flight and to "please sit".

Throughout my time in Russia I was to get used to the stock answer to every query, everywhere I went. Sit and wait! You learn, the hard way, the Soviet style of patience.

Four hours later I was led aboard a tiny aircraft, past a crowd of peasants all clamouring to get aboard. By this time it was twelve hours since I had last eaten or had anything to drink but I had struck a slight problem. I had no Russian roubles. You can't buy them outside the country and nobody was game to exchange my travellers cheques or American dollars inside. Result – a financial impasse. I decided, rumble tummied, I'd better hungrily bide my time and "sit and wait".

We'd only been in the air for seconds when my boots began to burn. Feeling gingerly down the wall of the aircraft to my toes, not wanting to create a fuss, I discovered the place where I was sitting right on the wing was red hot. How did I tell an aircraft full of passengers, who didn't speak a word of English, that we were on fire. How far was it to Leningrad? I didn't know. But I'll tell you what – I breathed a sign of relief when we landed safely.

One idiosyncrasy of Russian travel – you never know where you are going until you get there – even the name of your hotel. I was placed, I was told, in the Hotel Leningrad. You like it or lump it, but you certainly can't change or leave it as everything is paid in advance in the country where you obtained your visa.

The Hotel Leningrad was huge, enormous. It was like staying in London Airport with bedrooms. I timed it. It took five minutes to walk from the central elevator along the corridor to my room and there were ten similar floors. The room, which was tagged first class, was no more than a large, formica panelled cubicle with single bed, cupboards, a mirror, shoe cleaning brushes, a single blanket and a phone that you couldn't use without booking in advance.

I'd yet to meet the major hazard. Food. If you are not in a group or party you find it extremely difficult to get anything at all. Most of the tourists I met in Moscow or Leningrad were hungry. I began by trying at 11pm on the day of my arrival to get a cup of bedtime coffee. No roubles?

"I'm afraid," said the lady at the check-in desk politely, "you can't get roubles until the service bureau opens tomorrow at 9 am."

"Tomorrow?" I said bleakly.

Then, displaying a bit of British spirit, "But I'm hungry now."

"Sorry," said the lady looking even bleaker.

I retreated before she told me to "sit" again.

The next morning, feeling distinctly slimmer, I was in the service bureau queue when the doors opened. Breakfast, English style, however, was available only to the party bookings so I made do in a scruffy self-service joint with a cup of dishwater tea.

By the evening I was frantic and marched bravely into the restaurant. "Sorry," said the waitress, "Parties only." Desperate, I sat down at a table, banged my fist on the menu and, demanding "Supper – a la carte" stabbed a finger wildly at the Russian writing. I took a chance on anything. It turned out to be chicken noodle soup and ice cream with raspberry jam. It was the most welcome meal I had ever tasted.

Meanwhile I was doing my best to establish contact with the gerontologists. They were expecting me, I was informed, but where?

And then it happened! I was admiring a Russian doll in the tourist shop when Alexander Jacobovitch touched my shoulder. How could I know that within minutes this gracious, still handsome eighty year-old Russian gentleman would lift for me the veil on all the Leningrads of yesterday, today and yes, perhaps tomorrow.

When he was born there in 1896, Leningrad was then Petrograd, still the capital of all the Russias. The old gentleman now lives in

Mexico but, due to his advanced years, had been allowed by the authorities to return to revisit his birthplace.

There followed one of the most amazing stories I have ever heard, a story which gave me a glimpse of that other Leningrad of the historical past: the city behind the grim and stoic faces of the shabby men and women in the streets and the towering effigies of the soldiers of the Revolution, defying the competition of Capitalism with warning fists of black granite thrust high above the pavements.

Alexander Lapiner, as he is now called, gave me a glimpse instead of the magical city of his youth; a city of golden cupolas and misty spires; of a grey, gentle River Neva winding its way between ancient bridges and vast green parks which, in June, were heavy with the scent of lilacs; of palaces packed with some of the world's richest treasures and still peopled by the ghosts of the Tzars and the flying feet of gallant Cossack horsemen.

Alexander was a law student at Leningrad University in 1917 as Russia teetered on the brink of the revolutionary years of fighting and bloodshed to follow. At the time the city was dry and his father was running liquor into town in cardboard boxes. By the time of the Revolution later in 1917 and 1918, Alexander had joined the Revolutionary Army as an officer. Later when the White Russians took over he had to escape by night in a boat to Germany. And years of exile. Throughout the twenties and thirties he worked as a newspaper man in Germany and later became the European Public Relations Chief for the giant film corporation, Metro Goldwyn Meyer.

He was appointed to Prague and was at a farewell dinner in Warsaw when Hitler came marching in. He was one of only two survivors of the guests of that dinner, and as an employee of a top American company was shipped, a stateless person, to New York.

There followed years of hardship and stress. Alexander was employed on Broadway in New York. Finally he wrote to the boss of M.G.M. and started once again the long climb to the top. He was appointed to be P.R. boss of M.G.M. in South America. His proudest day was when he obtained his American Citizenship.

The only other survivor of that Warsaw dinner was flying to

meet him years later in South America when his plane crashed in dense jungle and he, too, was killed.

After relating his amazing story, my new found friend switched to the Russia of tomorrow. Hearing of my problems in contacting the gerontologists he offered to telephone for me and find out where my contact was to be made. He, of course, spoke fluent Russian. Then, realising my problems in finding interpreters he asked if I would like him to accompany me to the University to interpret for me during my interview. Which, is how I came to have an eighty year-old interpreter when I visited the oldest hospital in all Europe – an appropriate touch I thought.

Professor Dobrovolski was accompanied by a woman assistant, Professor Carsavetskaya, when we all gathered in the dark green office deep in the hospital of the Institute for Perfectionment of Doctors in Leningrad. It is, they explained, a hospital where many Russian doctors do Post Graduate training.

Everywhere we walked through the dank corridors, patients were sitting quietly, wearing striped pyjamas and dressing gowns. I couldn't help but recall Solzhenitsyn's famous book *Cancer Ward*.

Emphasising the importance to elderly people of being allowed to work and the value of making them feel integral parts of the community, the Professor said the Russians now have experimental parks for the aged.

"They are not old peoples' homes," he emphasised, "Those are of the past."

Instead, in Bachu, the northern capital of the region famous for oil, they have formed experimental parks. Here, old people live independently in their own homes around the perimeters of the park and each day they work, planting, making boxes or following their own craft.

Within the park are doctors of medicine and psychiatry, dentists, nurses and opticians who examine the old people on a regular basis.

In so many cases in the past, said the Professor, old people did not go to seek medical help when they needed it because they feared being put in old peoples' homes and losing their independence. In this way people could be helped into their old age feeling wanted and most important retaining their good health and independence.

The experiment was being repeated not only in other parts of Russia but also in other countries.

"What old people want is a moral standing in the community. This, we have discovered, from the sociological standpoint to be one of the most important factors in helping people to a healthy old age."

CHAPTER SEVEN

Hunza — Old Age On An Apricot Diet

"Hunza – it's a land of long life and good health. Our apricots hold the secret."

Prince Mohammed Ameen Khan,
Brother of the Mir of Hunza

They call the mysterious, remote Himalayan state of Hunza the very roof of the world. This hidden, secret valley ringed by the snow-capped peaks of some of the world's highest mountains is thought by many to be the real life Shangri-La – it was the inspiration for the idyllic valley of eternal youth in James Hilton's famous novel *Lost Horizon*.

Yet it is no fantasy, but scientific fact that the 35,000 inhabitants of this almost forgotten little kingdom are among the healthiest and most long lived in the world.

For over 800 years, until the start of this century, ruled over in feudal style by the Mir and his Royal ancestors, these fair skinned, blue eyed people, thought to descend from the Greek, Alexander the Great, were virtually cut off from the outside world.

Amid the snows and blue skies of their paradise in the sky, where time seems to stand still, they live to incredible ages – frequently well over 100, in almost perfect health – on a diet based on dried apricots and glacial mountain water laced with gold dust.

In a rugged hard working life style – 95% of Hunzacuts are farmers – they know little illness, no cancer, no heart disease, ulcers or nervous disorders and no tooth decay. They have only one doctor, no dentist and have never required a hospital in their history.

They live simply in stone and mud-daub houses, have little wealth, few possessions and, instead of currency, prefer to barter their goats, yaks and apricot trees. Consequently there are few pressures in their smiling, every day lives. Until the 1970s there were no police, no courts, no theft and no murder.

Scientists have said they do not regard it as entirely coincidental that the handful of spots in the world where people live exceptionally long lives are all high mountainous regions, virtually isolated from the rest of civilisation.

Hunza lies in one of the highest, most isolated, corners of Asia 8000 feet above sea level, on the borders of North-West Pakistan with Afghanistan and China. The lush green 107-mile long valley with its terraced slopes, tinkling streams and twinkling-eyed people is like some mountain mirage set amid this cruel perilous terrain, which once repelled even the advancing armies of Genghis Khan.

To get there I had to journey over one of the most breathtakingly beautiful, hair-raising routes known to man – over what adventurer-author Nicholas Monserrat has called "the mountains of fear."

Not so very long ago it was a 15-day perilous trek by pony or jeep over a boulder-strewn route which, in places, is literally lashed to the mountainside. Despite an ambitious new highway being built by Chinese and Pakistani soldiers – the area is not a top strategic military zone and requires a permit from the Pakistan Government to get there – the dangers for the traveller are only minimally less! If you don't fall over the side down a thousand foot precipice, you are likely to be hit on the head by a falling boulder.

I finally flew the 250 miles from Rawalpindi to Gilgit – a terrifying flight in itself, regarded by flying aces as one of the most dangerous in the world. At times our tiny, moth-like plane seemed only a wing-tip from the jagged white mountainsides as we flew over a never ending sea of serrated sugar icing peaks.

Hunza, where the last Mir was deposed by Ali Bhutto in 1974, was another death defying 68-mile journey by jeep. We were cut off on the way by four giant land slides.

The Hunzacuts welcome anyone who survives the ride. Today, they are a hard-working, simple race who give little thought to their long lives – 116 to 120 is the norm – and it has always been, so they say.

Apricots form the basis of the Hunza diet. They eat fresh apricots for three months of the year and the dried fruit for the rest of the year. A Hunzacut always has a pocketful of dried apricots to nibble and the biggest delicacy is the kernel. To throw away the stone is sacrilege in Hunza.

The late Mir's brother, Colonel Prince Aish Khan, told me: "We attribute our longevity to the apricots. Life is very simple in Hunza and the most important point is that we have no anxieties, no pressures."

Scientists say their longevity is almost certainly due to the apricot diet which consists mainly of fruit and vegetables. Meat is only eaten in the winter. They drink no tea or coffee. Instead they drink apricot juice and apricot soup and cook with apricot oil. Children chew apricot seeds, instead of sweets.

It is curious to note here that the controversial American cancer treatment, Laetrile B–17, discovered by San Francisco bio-chemist Dr Ernst T. Krebs Jnr., and said to actively retard or hold cancer at bay, is based on the apricot kernel. It is currently the subject of a U.S. Supreme Court case to try to get it de-restricted throughout America's 50 states.

Summing up Hunza's secret, Prince Mohammed Ameen Khan, brother of the present Mir, says: "Working hard, walking up and down steep hills each day, drinking icy glacial water and munching on dried apricots we keep in our pockets – that is the secret of our long life."

Certainly life is sweeter in Hunza.

CHAPTER EIGHT

Ecuador's Valley Of Eternal Youth

"I am not convinced that their life span – or ours – is limited to less than two hundred years."

Dr Donald Davies, University College, London

The most amazing Valley of Eternal Youth in the world is probably Vilcabamba – Indian for 'Sacred Valley' – 320 miles from the Ecuadorian capital of Quito.

In this incredible, forever smiling valley of youth, where its people live to 120 and beyond and women bear babies well into their fifties, today's children will almost certainly live to see the twenty-second century.

And in comparing the life style of the super centenarians of the world I feel it is interesting, if only to prove that the most important clue to longevity is the link between health, work and diet. Vilcabamba is a valley, where the sky is permanently blue, the air crisp and vital, an emerald valley of luscious fruits and vegetation, a Never-Never land of eternal youth where somehow it is always summer.

It is a valley of perfect peace; its inhabitants, who know none of the illnesses and killer diseases common to outside civilisation, live in an idyllic world completely lacking in stress or anxieties, in which there has never been a murder, rape or serious crime, where a man talks of his prowess in love at the age of 100, where at 121 a man complains he can no longer work more than a ten-hour day and women are proud of the fact that they work even harder than the men.

Around 2000 people live in the town dominated by a splendid

sandstone Roman Catholic church. Around it is a plaza with a park of tiny luxurious palms and sweet eucalyptus trees.

Another 3000 people live on the slopes around the town in farms and hamlets. The temperature is a warm, constant, 72 degrees Fahrenheit all the year round, which falls only a little at night, and the valley has no wild animals, snakes dangerous insects or even mosquitoes.

To reach the valley is a feat of endurance for those brave enough to try it – thirty-two miles of dirt track over gulleys, ravines and gorges from the nearest town of Loja.

The people live in adobe mud-brick homes with an earthen floor. A jumble of clay cooking pots holds their staple vegetables, herbs, hot peppers, and mint, sarandaja and orange leaves they brew daily into a refreshing drink like tea.

Wild and cultivated papayas grow like footballs, maize grows eight feet high and there are luxuriant growths of bananas, sweet corn, barley, grapes, tomatoes, oats and sugar cane. There for the picking, too, are the sweetest apples, peaches, oranges, guavas, mangoes, bulging, black raspberries, watermelons, loquats and tangerines.

Their staple diet is cheese, fruit and vegetables. According to the priest, Father Francisco Bravo, – this is the reason people are so healthy.

"They eat sparingly and they have real peace. That is why they live so long."

The daily calorie intake of the Vilcabambas is 1700 calories. Their most popular staple vegetable is a white root, called yuka, which, when boiled, becomes very like a floury potato. Dr Alex Comfort, author of the best-selling *The Joy Of Sex* is an expert on gerontology and the problems of ageing. He says, "People in Vilcabamba don't get blood vessel diseases because they do not eat a lot of animal fats. You see fat people in most cultures but here there is virtually no obesity." There is no baldness either.

A zoologist from the Gerontology Department of London's University College, Dr Donald Davies, who was invited by the Ecuador Government to organise studies of the people who lived to 120 and beyond, said many of the old people were still producing blood cells at 120.

He suspected their excellent circulation was connected to muscular development. "These are mountain people and their calf muscles are so huge they are virtually second hearts," he said.

It is fascinating to note the marked similarity between the Caucasians, Hunzacuts and Vilcabambas. All have a similar low calorie fruit and vegetable, low fat, diet; all have a stress and anxiety free life style; in each case retirement is unknown and a man works hard every day of his life; there is no obesity, heart disease, cancer and mental illness and the common infectious diseases of our society seem to be unknown.

However, apart from cutting down on our calorie intake, working like trojans until we drop dead and moving our homes lock stock and barrel to the high mountains, what else can *we* do in the big fight?

CHAPTER NINE

Cell Therapy

"Nobody can make you younger; you cannot add years to your life but you can add life to your years."

Dr Joachim Stein, Vice-President,
The International Society for Research on Cell Therapy

Everywhere I've been, since I first admitted to a friend that I intended to find out the truth about rejuvenation, people have been looking at me rather as if I were the two-headed lady in the fairground.

But, half-amused half-intrigued, they always come up with exactly the same questions whether young, old, believers or sceptics: "Yes, but do any of these treatments really work?"

And, more specifically: "Have you tried any of them yourself?"

I didn't set out on my travels with the idea of being some sort of human guinea pig. I have far too much regard for my own looks and good health for that. But I did agree to try cell therapy – today's most popular and successful treatment in the battle against age.

And while rejuvenators still can't turn back the clock and transform a seventy year-old into a forty year-old or make a fifty-five year-old look twenty again, we can still fairly effectively manage to look a good ten to twenty years younger than our actual or chronological age and keep that way during the rest of our life span as well as retaining much of the vitality and libido of youth.

Cell therapy – rejuvenation, or as doctors practising it prefer to call it, revitalisation – as a result of injections of cells of unborn lambs – is still one of the most controversial treatments in modern medicine. But it can no longer be classed as revolutionary.

Since it was discovered by the legendary youth doctor, Professor Dr Paul Niehans, over forty years ago, around two million people have received cell therapy treatment.

Niehans alone treated over forty thousand patients up to his death in 1971 at the ripe old age of ninety, and none of his patients ever died as a direct result of having received the injections.

To find out all there is to know about cell – or more accurately, cellular therapy, its correct name – I traced it to its source in Switzerland, tracked down one of the leading world authorities, Dr Joachim Stein, at a medical congress in Berlin and later flew to Germany again to see the famous laboratories in Heidelberg in the Black Forest where the cells are extracted, processed and freeze-dried to be sent out all over the world.

I talked to doctors practising the treatment as far afield as Bavaria in Germany, Britain, the Fiji Islands, and in Noumea in the French tropical islands of New Caledonia in the South Pacific, where I tried cell therapy first hand.

What exactly is cell therapy? In simple terms it is the subcutaneous injection into the human body of hundreds of thousands of cells and minute cell unions.

It is estimated that within our body some fifty million cells die every second and the same number are replaced. However, when we are sick or prematurely aged the quality and number of that replacement falls off and the cells that are replaced are imperfect. For example, when the parts of a motor car are being manufactured from a mould or template, thousands of identical parts keep on being reproduced. But if there was a dent or damage to one of those templates, the part similarly being reproduced would also be damaged.

It is the same in the human body. When a part such as the liver or heart or bone marrow has damage through toxins, infection, disease, nicotine or alcohol, then the cells will not remould to the original quality and standard. However, cells from unborn animals are still completely undamaged. Through cell therapy the damaged organ or tissue is said to receive a new template from which to rebuild the corresponding organ.

Basically we can outline two main effects from cell therapy.

Firstly, general revitalisation or regeneration which the experts say can only be obtained through cellular injections from placenta or testes. Secondly, the organ specific effect. This may sound technical but for the layman it simply means that injections or, as doctors call them, implants of cells from the different organs act on the corresponding organ in the patient's body, ie. heart on heart, kidney on kidney. How these are transported to the correct or specific spot I will explain in more detail later.

Next you are going to ask: why are sheep and lambs used in preference to other animals or indeed humans? To start with animal cells are the same biochemical structure as those of the human organism. Sheep are preferred, in particular, because of their health and resistance to disease and the ease of keeping them in isolated flocks. The reason for using the foetus to obtain most of the cells is mainly because in the unborn animal cells are still completely sterile, being well protected in the womb. Secondly, and more particularly, the foetus does not have its immune defence system activated at this time to fight against bacteria and virus. The new born has no antibodies of its own, using those of the mother, and, therefore, its antigen qualities are extremely low. Thus there is less likelihood of rejection by the host organ in the patient's body after the cell injections.

Where is cell therapy available? Today cell therapy is available at many rejuvenation and revitalisation clinics all over the world. Many medically qualified doctors practice the technique, which they believe to be beneficial in the treatment of many of the diseases of ageing as well as retaining youth.

Among the many diseases cell therapy is said to have successfully helped to alleviate are sex and menstrual disorders, obesity caused by gland disorders, impotence in men, premature ageing and degenerative diseases of the vascular system, chronic rheumatism, arthrosis, degenerative diseases of the heart, kidneys, lungs and stomach and chronic digestive disorders.

It is also being used today with great success in the treatment of mongolism. In West Germany, for example, by far the most liberal, medically, in its views of treatments to prevent ageing, it is claimed by the German Society For Cell Therapy that there are around six thousand registered medical practitioners using cell therapy.

This is by far the largest number in any single country of the world but the freeze-dried fresh cells are officially exported from Switzerland and Germany to about forty-six countries.

Others like the United States, with far more stringent drug and customs laws, do not allow the cells to be imported for clinical use. However, patients anxious to receive the treatment have found many ways round restrictions. Packages marked "Gift Only" containing the cell ampoules are frequently mailed from the European laboratories to Mexico and the Bahamas to then be re-routed to clients, many of them doctors, in the U.S.

Until comparatively recently, however, the film stars, rich and famous, potentates, royalty and heads of state who flocked to Niehan's clinic in Switzerland managed to keep the treatment almost exclusively to themselves. Since the 1930's they travelled in cloak and dagger secrecy to Niehan's expensive clinic, a giant sugar icing chalet on the shores of Lake Geneva near Montreux, believing they would be kept in the pink of their youth and health by the injections from freshly slaughtered unborn lambs.

In the early years, to be rich and famous was just about the only way you'd gain access to the clinic run by the proud and autocratic Prussian surgeon. Niehans has always maintained a rigid button-lipped silence on the subject of the clients who entered his shuttered chalet, but the rumours of the famous who went there multiplied over the years along with his fame. The clients pounding the route to his door willing to pay $1,500 fee for his injections read more and more like an international *Who's Who*.

Marlene Dietrich, in her 70's and still one of the world's most glamorous women, attributes her youthful looks to Niehan's method. The Duchess of Windsor, Sir Charles Chaplin, the Shah of Iran, Cary Grant, Picasso, Gloria Swanson, Sir Winston Churchill, President Kennedy, Kirk Douglas, the Emperor of Japan, Somerset Maugham, Noel Coward, Christian Dior, Konrad Adenauer and even President De Gaulle himself have all been persistently rumoured to have been clients, and although few ever admitted it, none of them has ever denied it.

One of Niehan's colleagues told me that once he recalled seeing three kings, one of whom was Emperor Haille Selassie, all at Montreux, unknown to each other, being treated at the same time.

Niehan's most famous client of all was Pope Pius XII, who first put the seal of respectability on the treatment and rocketed Niehans into the multi-million dollar success story he became.

In 1920, Paul Niehans, then thirty-eight, was a successful young surgeon. A doctor of theology before he turned to medicine, he was reliably said to be the grandson of King Frederick III of Germany and a Princess of Furstenberg. Because the Princess was not of equal birth with the Hohenzollerns they were unable to marry officially and the Emperor (father of the last Kaiser) later married Princess Victoria of England, daughter of Queen Victoria.

Whether or not Niehans personally had the bearing of a royal aristocrat, throughout his life he remained cool and aloof, suffering no fools. Nor did the many, who tried to blacken his reputation or topple him from his millionaire pedestal by labelling him as a quack and charlatan, appear even to halt the tall, distinguished-looking doctor in his controversial route which took over his earlier orthodox medical career. He believed firmly in what he was doing even if he didn't begin to understand the real medical reasons beneath the success of his methods.

However, the idea of cell implantation had been buzzing around the minds of physicians for centuries. In the earliest medical writings known to man, specifically the Papyrus of Ebers, mention is made of preparations made from animal and human organs. Similar mention was made by Aristotle.

Hippocrates – the man on whom the medical hippocratic oath is based – spoke of skin transplantation from animals to man. And, as early as the beginning of the 16th century Paracelsus, the famous doctor of the Middle Ages, is known to have stated: "Simila similibus curantur: like cures like." Although it is certain he could not then have possibly known the full importance and implications of what he was advocating.

From the time of Hunter in England of the 1770's and in 1849, Berthold in Gottingen, studies were made and established on the effect of implanting testes in castrated roosters.

In 1889 Dr Charles Edouard Brown-Sequard, then seventy-two, son of an Irish-American sea captain and a French woman, became even better known when he experimented by injecting himself with an extract from the testicles of dogs. Brown-Sequard told a gathering of academics in Paris that after three injections he was able to put the clock back thirty years. He was, of course, referring to his renewed and vigorous sex life – but it appears the effects were only transient. Unfortunately the newly energetic doctor went overboard and even built a machine to pulverise bulls' testicles to produce a magical revitalisation liquid, which thousands of people rushed to try.

Sadly, at this point his dyed-in-the-wool, more orthodox colleagues turned their back on him and his ballyhoo, and another dream of eternal youth died.

If we are looking for the very beginnings of cell therapy and the first ideas of transplanting foreign cells from one organism into another, we should include blood transfusion. It was as long ago as 1667 that Jean Baptiste Denis first transfused blood into a man.

But it was Landsteiner's revolutionary discovery of the major blood groups in 1900, which won him the Nobel Prize in Medicine, that opened the way to allow blood transfusions to become the first safe form of cell implantation.

During the First World War (1914-18) blood transfusions revolutionised military medicine, saving many thousands of lives following some of the bloodiest fighting in history.

Subsequently, doctors discovered how to freeze rare blood types invaluable for use during the Vietnam War.

Niehans began to experiment implanting cells by intramuscular injection in the 1920's. To start with he called his theory "Tissular Transplantation". In 1927 he injected the eosinophilic cells of the anterior lobe of the pituitary gland from calves into a young human dwarf. It is said that the experiment resulted in the dwarf increasing his height by 32 centimetres.

Niehans' meteoric rise to world fame, however, happened more or less as a result of an accident.

Around this period, scientists everywhere were becoming increasingly intrigued in the idea of transplanting tissue from one creature into another. The first serious seeds of interest were being sown in endocrinology, the study of hormones and glandular transplants. The man in vogue during the roaring 'twenties was the mysterious and eccentric Russian born surgeon, Professor Serge Voronoff, who had caught the imagination of people everywhere with his monkey gland transplants, the infamous monkey glands as they were to become – the treatment that was in effect to put gerontology and all its researchers into disrepute for several decades.

At the time, however, Voronoff was enjoying a blaze of publicity. With the sort of fervor which surrounded Christian Barnard's heart transplants in 1967, the Russian scientist in his forbidding Chateau Grimaldi on the Italian Riviera was acclaimed for his success in pioneering the transplant of pieces of testicle from chimpanzees into male patients.

Unfortunately for Voronoff, he failed to heed the warnings of other contemporary researchers on the dangers of transmitting disease into his patients along with the glands. When some of his male clients developed V.D. the monkey gland era ended, not surprisingly, in a wave of nausea, horror and disgust which is still recalled today.

Niehans, however, was intrigued by the concept of gland transplants. Always an unusual young man he was a friend of Voronoff and had watched him operate. It was quite natural, therefore, on April Fools's Day, April 1, 1931 at a clinic in Lausanne that it was Niehans who was called in to do an emergency operation to carry out what was initially intended to be a simple parathyroid gland transplant. After all, he was one of the few doctors of the moment known to have any knowledge of the technique.

For Niehans it turned out to be the occasion that was to set the course for the rest of his life . . .

A young Swiss doctor was operating on a woman patient suffering from goitre. Accidentally, however, he snipped through the adjacent parathyroid glands producing a serious condition called iatrogenic tetany in which the patient's calcium level falls, resulting in cramp-like muscular spasms. Unless emergency treatment was carried out immediately it seemed inevitable that the woman would die.

The doctors immediately thought of trying a transplant of the parathyroid glands from an animal but the one man who could help them was, of course, Paul Niehans.

By the time the doctor had received the emergency call and stopped on the way to the clinic to slaughter a calf steer and remove the needed glands, the young woman patient was near to death.

Once at her side, Niehans realised, as she went into convulsions, that it was unlikely she could survive the surgical operation. In desperation, anxious to save the woman and his colleague's reputation, Niehans made an instant decision. He cut up the parathyroid glands into minute slices, taking great care not to mash the cells and put them into a solution. He then placed the lot in a large hypodermic syringe and to the horror of the watching doctors plunged it into the woman's breast muscle.

To everyone's amazement – apart perhaps from Niehans – the tetany disappeared almost at once and the woman recovered. Not only that, but she lived another thirty years to die well into her nineties.

A strange introduction, perhaps, but cell therapy had begun.

In 1951 Niehans is said to have been consulted by the British Royal Family when King George VI was dying of lung cancer.

However, his most famous patient was undoubtedly Pope Pius XII. The Pontiff was 78 and very frail when the rejuvenator was first called to the Papal bedside at the Pope's summer palace at Castall Gandolfo, in 1954. He was suffering from hiccups. Later that year when the Pope was again seriously ill and his own Vatican doctors were near despair, Niehans was called in once more. This time he did in fact administer cell therapy, using specially prepared freeze dried cells.

However, to the embarrassment of the Pope's own doctors who had failed to help, the Pope recovered, cured by what science persisted in calling simply "quack medicine". Whatever the reason for his recovery, the Pope was convinced it was due to Niehans and put the final accolade on the treatment by publicly acclaiming it. Later he further astounded scientists by awarding him the Chair in the Pontifical Academy vacated by the death of the man who discovered penicillin, Sir Alexander Fleming. From then on Niehans' fame knew no bounds, although many said he was ripping off the many people desperate for youth by charging such exorbitant prices. But those who wanted his treatment were only too happy to pay.

Niehans had many disciples, men who worked closely with him – like his successors at La Prairie Clinique, in Clarens-Montreux, the head of which is now Dr B. Bovet, and many others who took his principles and determined to carry out the vital task which Niehans, in his arrogance, ignored: to prove to the scientific world just how and why cell therapy works so that it can be accepted as conventional medicine instead of remaining, as it has for so many years, on the fringe.

One such man is Dr Joachim Stein, the tall and distinguished German scientist, who has devoted most of his working lifetime to the advance of cell therapy and who today, ranks as a world authority on the technique. He is also a Vice President of both the International Society for Research in Cell Therapy and the German Society for Cell Therapy, both with headquarters in Frankfurt am Main. The former is a body of over forty university professors working together in the fields of anatomy, physiology, biochemistry and tissue culture and the latter exists to exchange information and experiences among member practitioners.

In 1954, following five years of preliminary experiments by Niehans, Dr Stein successfully began freeze drying or lyophilising fresh cells from the lamb foetus and other young animals so that they could be preserved and exported easily to any country in the world and indeed used months later by physicians. These are now produced commercially under the name of Siccacells.

Today, mainly thanks to Stein's efforts, patients thousands of miles apart can receive the revitalising injections obtained from around seventy different tissues and organs ranging from the liver and heart to placenta, testes, spleen, kidney, hypothalmus, bone marrow, thymus and even the brain.

At the famous Cybila Laboratories in Heidelberg of which he is head, I went to see how the cells are obtained and prepared in one of the most dramatic and, if you are squeamish – gruesome factories in the world.

Personally, I found it fascinating.

The streamlined, attractive and modern two storey, ice-cool blue building six miles outside Heidelberg, the ancient university town in the heart of Germany's Black Forest region, fulfilled one of Niehans' greatest dreams. He provided much of the capital to build it so that his work could be carried out world wide. From the entrance hall a spiral staircase leads upwards to offices, the conference room where doctors from all over the world come to listen to Dr Stein and his colleagues, in the boardroom, where a black and white portrait of the great rejuvenator who started it all, dominates one wall.

Below are a labyrinth of sterile white corridors, laboratories, operating theatres, packing and despatch rooms and an abattoir where the tiny lambs are delivered by Caesarean section operation just a few days before the expected date of their birth.

Dr Stein with his precisely clipped German accent – he studied medicine in Berlin – is handsome and boyish looking, the ideal advocate for cell therapy. At sixty-two he was just starting serious mountaineering as a hobby and he jogs up the steeply wooded mountainside around Heidelberg, the grey stone town which lies sleepily in its tree shrouded bowl, every morning of his life.

His leather-topped desk, I noted, was precisely neat and orderly just like the man. A cream and brown leather-covered telephone, a golden rose, a pottery rabbit with enormous ears (surely, it should have been a lamb?), and two red roses in a green glass vase.

Seating himself at the head of the giant polished wood boardroom table he prepared to tell me in detail exactly how the famous cell injections are obtained and prepared.

The flock of 2500-3000 specially bred sheep used by the laboratories are kept in isolation in hilly grazing country about twenty-five miles from the Heidelberg factory. The sheep are protected carefully, fenced in away from pollution, traffic and urban civilisation. Every detail on each donor animal is carefully recorded, its antecedents, its medical history and each sheep is earmarked with its number.

They are controlled by veterinary surgeons both from the

Cybila Laboratories and the University Veterinary Hygiene Institution who visit the flock and take blood, urine and stool samples every six weeks.

The pregnant ewes carry their young normally for a gestation period of five months, and after three and a half months they are moved from the country to a quarantine station adjoining the laboratory. There, under completely sterile conditions the ewe spends the remainder of her time in waiting in pampered comfort. During this period the sheep is put through endless bacteriological, serological and clinical tests to ensure that all the diseases which could be transferred from an animal to a patient have been excluded.

There are altogether around thirty-six different zoonoses or possible diseases that could be transmitted, although only twenty-seven actually in Germany, and the scientists take the utmost care to see that every chance of this happening is eliminated.

Says Doctor Stein: "One pregnant ewe up to the moment she is slaughtered here has cost between DM25,000 ($1316/£641) to DM38,000 ($1473/£717) in laboratory tests. That is one of the reasons why cell therapy is still expensive." A single combination set of three to ten different types of cells, one treatment for a patient, costs anything from DM233 ($122/£60) to DM473 ($249/£122) a set.

If they could find a method of sterilising without denaturing or damaging the cells by changing their biochemical composition then it would be far cheaper to the patient.

Nothing I have previously seen prepared me for the quarantine stables. Row upon row of caged rats, white mice, guinea pigs and rabbits all living in sterile, air conditioned compartments. The walls are pale green and the straw in the areas reserved for the sheep was so clean you'd swear it must have been through a washing machine.

The air is filtered and the keeper who looks after the animals is the only person allowed to have contact with them apart from the vets. He has to change his own clothes for sterile clothing, wears a surgical mask and has to wash his hands and wear rubber gloves.

The animals are fed a normal diet but the food, all sterilised and rich in proteins, is prepared specially for experimental animals. I even tasted some myself – it was rather like liquorice.

I said these must be the cleanest sheep anywhere in the world. Dr Stein agreed, but pointed out that they were just normal, sturdy, sound country sheep.

After four weeks in quarantine the sheep is shorn and then is moved in a specially closed vehicle to the laboratories' own slaughter house.

As we passed through the quarantine stable and peered through the double glass windows, I was amazed to see three tiny lambs, obviously alive and kicking, nestling to their mother's side. Apparently they cheated the scientists by arriving two days early. I had to admit a sneaking feeling of delight that they and their mother had escaped death, this time round anyway, and would soon be returning to the fresh air, the fields and the rest of the flock!

When we arrived back in the main laboratory building I was told to abandon my street clothes and climb into surgical gown, gloves, mask and clumpy rubber operating boots. Then, looking like something from outer space, I flip-flopped my way awkwardly towards the slaughter house and operating theatre.

The sparkling cleanliness of the abattoir would have put many a kitchen to shame. It was pristine with scrubbed tiled floors, sealed doors and a metal crisscross of pulleys and overhead trolleys on which the animals are suspended.

The ewe is at this point washed with a body-warm sterilising solution to kill any germs in the fleece and is then anaesthetised by electric shock. The animal is bled by opening the carotides or arteries in the neck, in order to extract as much blood as possible from the placenta while the heart is still beating.

The ewe is finally covered with a sterile cloth and the belly shaved and disinfected in the preparation for a Caesarean section operation to remove the complete womb from the mother.

Although the ewe is dead by this time the foetuses – there are usually two baby lambs within the womb – are still alive. They have sufficient oxygen and nutrition to go on living for a further twenty minutes.

Immediately the womb is removed it is placed in a double sterile container and rushed to the operating theatre. The womb is passed through a hatch or lock into an inner, completely germ-free sterile compartment which Dr Stein describes as a glove box. It is completely air tight and has high air pressure so that if a mistake has been made the air can only pass outwards, not in. The whole box is disinfected by formalin and is inside the operating room.

The surgeon and his assistants work through two glove holes like cuffed gauntlets and only their sterile rubber gloved hands come into contact with the foetus.

Quickly, within five to six minutes, they remove all the main organs and with curved scissors cut the tissue into small cubes and place them in a suspension solution. The pieces are then cut even finer with a special angled chopping knife until the pieces are no more than 0.3 millimetres in length.

If sufficient speed is used and the utmost care taken at this juncture, subsequent microscope tests show that no more than 10% of the cells are destroyed.

The pieces of each organ must then be placed in separate stainless steel sterile containers after which they can be moved from the glove box into the adjoining deep freezing room. Here the cells are deep frozen within a fraction of a second to minus 85 degrees centigrade or celsius.

Once the cells are in this deep frozen state no further chemical or enzymal changes or reactions can take place. The organs are now placed in a lyophilisation chamber, and here in a very high vacuum during the next thirty-six hours or less the humidity is extracted and the cells freeze dried to a residual humidity of about 0.6%. Some "structural" water is left in order to retain the chemical balance of the organs.

Next this dried material, again in a glove box, is cut up and passed through a sieve to eliminate all the connective tissue and arteries so that only the cells are left.

At this point the fragments of tissue are a light yellowish-grey in colour. They are fed into ampoules and then go through a second drying procedure in a vacuum to restore the optimal residual moisture of 0.6% again. After a few hours the ampoules are sealed under vacuum. Any one ampoule could contain anything between eight hundred million and one billion cells. It is known that it can be kept in this phial not under refrigeration and even in tropical climates for anything up to eighteen years and still be used for injection without any deterioration in the cells.

Even now, Dr Stein told me, the tests for sterility are not yet over. About every tenth ampoule of each production batch is sent to the University Institute of Hygiene. Here, they check for about six weeks for sterility as some slow developing germs can only be detected up to that length of time.

At the same time, samples from the same lot are being injected into experimental rats and mice for further tests. Only at the end of that time is a batch given a germ free certificate and passed.

In further health controls in Germany even organs from the mother ewe are dissected and examined by the German State Health Authorities in Heidelberg.

Said Dr Stein: "This is really the strictest, tightest system of control you could imagine. We can guarantee the sterility of the lyophilised cells and also that they are absolutely unchanged."

In order to prepare the lyophilised cells for injection all the doctor has to do is to combine the cells with a special solution – a Pannett-Compton solution – either in the ampoule or syringe, and after thirty seconds to one minute it is ready for injection into the patient.

Which leads me to the next part of the story – how I had cell therapy . . .

The Qantas jet dropped gently towards the palm fringed holiday island of French New Caledonia in the South Pacific. I glanced with curiosity at my fellow passengers. Which of them, I wondered, were heading for more than just an ordinary holiday in the sun? How many of them were using this package tour as a cover while they secretly spent their dollars shopping for youth?

One week earlier the first cell therapy clinic in the southern hemisphere had quietly opened its doors in Noumea, but already the local people were buzzing with excitement over the prospect of cashing in on a world famous Island of Eternal Youth.

The Clinic was being run by a young, handsome French doctor

with its headquarters in the plushy and expensive Château Royale Hotel. With its adjoining Casino and curving white beaches shaded by coconut palms, I couldn't think of a more idyllic spot to search for renewed youth and perhaps an exciting new sex life in the sun!

The people waiting for their baggage in Tontouta Airport looked much the same as any other crowd of international travellers. I was thrust into an airport car with a motley cross section. A blonde woman with brassy hair and a much younger boyfriend; a middle-aged woman who had combed her hair throughout the entire two and a half hour flight from Sydney and an older woman artist with an extremely loud voice.

Were any of these the Cell People? I couldn't hazard a guess and if they were they weren't admitting it – certainly not to me, anyway.

I've discovered that, in general, patients undergoing youth treatment are notoriously loath to talk about it. Perhaps they are frightened other people will laugh or think them vain, or even worse, cruelly accuse them of being mutton dressed as lamb?

Typical was the way in which, during the weeks before the clinic officially opened, top showbiz and television personalities had been flying in from Australia with the same hush-hush hysteria, wearing dark glasses, using assumed names and hiding away in their hotel rooms while they underwent the treatment.

Since then hundreds of ordinary men and women of all ages had been flocking in, anxious to tap the fountain of youth themselves. We all met for the first time that evening at an informal briefing session at which the doctor was to tell us all about the treatment. I noted with satisfaction that brassy hair and the woman artist were among us!

We gathered in a large, cool, all white suite on the sixth floor of the hotel. It had white vinyl furnishings, white carpet – a huge local tapestry dominating one wall. The doctor, I recall, with a touch of typical French élan, also wore white – a white linen suit with matching soft leather shoes.

Quietly in his soft French accent he led us through the outline principles of cell therapy. And, typically, most of us on the eve of our first youth treatment were apprehensive and unsure.

The next morning we were instructed to turn up at his modern surgery in downtown Noumea for a health check. I must say here that, in general, most cell therapists do seem to take tremendous care in checking out the patient's medical history before treatment in order to give the most beneficial combination of injections.

Most of us, in fact, had already attended a medical with a fully qualified doctor in our home town before leaving and these records had been forwarded to the doctor to be consulted at the time of treatment. He was anxious to know full medical background – aches, pains, operations, childhood illnesses. Any problems?

Finally, I got the OK. Report for therapy at 2pm.

By the time I arrived I was in an agony of apprehension. Climbing onto the doctor's couch I waited, tense as a tiger, for the five syringes of frothing, pink cells to be thrust into my backside. Like darts into a pincushion the quivering needles pinged into my posterior and, closing my eyes and clenching my muscles from top to toe, I waited for the youth jabs that were going to keep me looking young.

I have to admit I am a coward when it comes to anything that might have a vestige of pain attached, and originally I had no intention of undergoing cell therapy personally. Oh no! I was just going to talk to others braver than I about their experiences. But by their conspiracy of silence I found the only way of getting the facts was to do it myself. What a martyr! But I needn't have worried. When it comes down to it, it is all very painless and simple.

The five injections I received, two in one side, three in the other, injected subcutaneously into the facia of the hip muscle, were for general revitalisation, all that is necessary if you are still young and healthy as in my case. They contained placenta for general toning, foetal thymus to help in fighting infection, liver cells, hypothalmus and vertebrae bone marrow cells aimed at improving a general back tension.

The only slight after effect I felt was a general ache in the muscles in the injection area and a slight tiredness that night and the next day. The doctor told me to relax for two to three days, not to do anything strenuous and not to smoke or drink alcohol after the jabs. Some patients told me they felt fantastic immediately after the injections, which is quite general, although the full effect is not normally noticed until two to three months afterwards.

Doctors tell me they consider a woman should have cell therapy ideally from the age of twenty-five onwards. However, if she starts by thirty, before wrinkling and deterioration begins, she can expect to keep ahead and keep in peak condition looking ten to twenty years younger than her age for the rest of her life!

Doctors vary in their view of how often injections should be repeated. It depends very much on the energy and the general health of the patient. But normally people return for a booster course about every three to five years although Dr Stein, says one set of injections has stood him in good stead ever since!

The doctor in Noumea, whose name I have been unable to use because of strict French medical ethics, said he believed that while cell therapy is not allowed in countries like Australia and the U.S. it would be available everywhere within the next ten years. "Its benefits are enormous," he told me.

How did I feel after having the treatment? In the weeks immediately after, I must admit I personally didn't feel or look particularly different. However, in recent months I have been full of an energy I never had before. But I do wish people would stop telling me I look great for seventy!

The most controversial question of all, which medicos argue in refusing to accept cell therapy as conventional medicine, is how the cells reach the corresponding specific organs in the human body.

Dr Stein explains it this way: the human body is a community state containing something like fifteen trillion cells – a fantastic number at which we can only guess. In one cubic millimetre of blood, that's the size of the head of a needle, there are about 4.5 million red blood cells. Every cell in our body is a living, complete unit.

It has been pointed out already that cell therapy is of use only in the treatment of degenerative diseases – that means the consequences of wear and tear or the results of infectious diseases, alcohol, nicotine and pollution such as car exhausts. All these factors damage the biological structure of the cells. It's like a car in which the pistons are worn out.

Every one of these cells in our bodies constantly breaks down and rebuilds its own proteins. The broken down proteins go into the blood as amino acids and are excreted. For example, in one hundred days the liver, which is one of the most active metabolic organs, exchanges its substance completely – it is made up of completely renewed cells.

However, at the same time that an organ is being broken down it is rebuilding and if it is damaged it will rebuild with the same imperfections. So a person with cirrhosis of the liver, for example, will retain a similarly damaged liver. So you get identical reduplication.

When new cells are implanted into the human body through cell therapy they are each absorbed by a phagoctye – white blood cells which have the capacity to eat up materials like alien foreign particles. For example, when you have an infection in your finger from bacteria it is the phagocytes from the blood which come along, swallow them up and then excrete them.

This is what happens to the cells. Phagocytes break down the proteins in the cells, dissolving them with enzymes and transport the remnants to the corresponding or specific organ. The important part that is left is the organ specific material vital to the rebuilding of the new cells.

How do scientists know this? Dr Stein explains: "We found out in investigations by marking cells with isotopes. We injected isotopes into pregnant sheep. Then they moved into the foetus without damaging the foetus. We then injected these cells and tissues into other animals so we could follow with a geiger counter the way the cells went. At the beginning we had to use isotope elements like phosphorus, iodine, sulphur, but now amino acids, the building material of the protein, can be tagged. We found out that the organ specific material kidney or heart or spleen, really does end up in the correct corresponding specific organ."

For this reason it is no good giving cell therapy to a perfectly normal healthy man or woman with normal functions. You cannot after all stimulate a normal organ to over-function. But once the body is on the verge of starting the downward degenerative run to old age and disease, from twenty-five onwards, then and only then can results be obtained.

Here, for your guidance, is a list of the conditions and diseases which have been found to have been helped by cell therapy.

Dr Stein points out, however, that cell therapy is only used for degenerative diseases. It is never used to treat infections or inflammatory diseases. The conditions it can help alleviate are as follows:

General revitalisation
Arteriosclerosis
Cardiosclerosis
Menopause Syndrome
Peripheral perfusion disorders
Chronic osteoarthritis
Arthrosis deformans
Neurodystonia
Chronic peptic ulcer
Chronic non-osbstructive emphysema
Chronic indigestion
Chronic hepotopathy
Parkinson's Disease

Dr Stein is, however, honest. Cell therapy is not 100% effective. Out of several million patients the percentage success rate is good to very good for 67-68%; moderate results for 10-15%, and for the rest there is no noticeable result at all.

One of the problems with cell therapy is to discover a reputable qualified practitioner. To find out the names of doctors/clinics using cell therapy in your immediate country or area of the world you can write either to The Scientific Advisory Service of Cybila in Heidelberg or to The International Society for Research of Cell Therapy in Frankfurt. The addresses are:

Cybila,
Wissenschaftlicher Beratungsdienst,
Cytobiologische Laboratorien GmbH,
Hauptstrabe 20,
D-6900 Heidelberg 1,
West Germany

Internationale Forschungsgesellschaft für Zelltherapie,
Blanchardstrabe 22,
D-6000 Frankfurt am Main 90,
West Germany
Telephone: 0611/776620

CHAPTER TEN

Body Servicing

"Can it be now said – you are only young – TWICE?"
London Sunday Mirror

Peter Stephan, Britain's leading youth specialist, offers a top to toe method of revitalising and rejuvenating his thousands of patients – Body Servicing. For the last fifteen years, ever since he took over his father's practice at the age of only twenty-one, Stephan's name had been synonymous with cell therapy in Britain. But today he describes his latest methods as a serious extension of Niehans' original ideas – a modernised up-dated version which gives the whole body system new vigour and health. He serves it up under the name of Cell Revitalisation Therapy. Patients who knock at Stephan's door just off Harley Street in London frequently tell him: "I know you can't give me the world – but maybe you can give me the moon."

Stephan says that more than half his patients are from outside the United Kingdom and he sees well over one thousand people a year. Most of them come complaining about stiff joints, the menopause and their looks (the women), sexual difficulties (the men), or inability to escape from constant anxieties or nagging stress. Others are so physically and mentally tired they can no longer sleep, their digestion suffers, they have headaches, wandering back aches and various other niggling pains for which no reasons can be pin-pointed, but which nevertheless make life a misery.

Certainly, most of them come looking for a miracle, but Stephan doesn't lead them up the garden path.

He is an articulate, chubby-faced Yorkshireman who you feel at once will call a spade a spade; who talks such basic commonsense you can't help but like him.

What he does say of the treatment he offers at prices between $1000/£500 and $1200/£600 for a two week course is this: "The treatment is valuable – it does work, patients do respond and they do feel better, they do live longer and they have a much better attitude to life.

"Maybe one day we will be able to offer to make someone fifty years younger. But right now, what we are offering as a form of treatment is to slow down the ageing process and balance the system to help people function better mentally and physically throughout their entire life span, whether that is sixty, seventy-two or ninety-six. They won't find themselves suddenly senile."

Certainly, many of them only a few weeks after treatment report finding themselves as springy as new born lambs. Stephan believes the ageing process will slow down even more if a man or woman undergoes his treatment as young as twenty-five or thirty, as in normal cell therapy.

Stephan looks prosperous, which he is, white polo neck sweater, lots of gold jewellery, English gentlemen's cavalry twill suit. He admits he has made a fortune out of cell therapy and enjoyed the luxury side benefits – the country mansion, the Rolls convertible with the PS1 number plates.

But he says all the showy signs of extravagance are now behind him. Today he wriggles uncomfortably when you try to pigeonhole his profession. He no longer wants to be known as a cell therapist, he says, although he personally has given between fifty to sixty thousand cell injections over the years. Now he says he is far more interested in the scientific side of his work and in employing laboratories to document its value indisputably to the medical profession.

At present, the researches Stephan is helping finance are aimed in one direction: to find an ultimate youth treatment that has no side effects at all, one that doctors everywhere will be able to use in their own surgery without question.

I went to see Peter Stephan at his London mews consulting rooms at 27 Harley Place, W1, just a stride away from the very heart of London's snob medical consultant belt.

The cobbled street was quiet in the summer afternoon heat as I waited for an answer to my ring. The private secretary with the terribly Oxford English accent was kindness itself as she asked me to wait. Stephan, the dynamo, arrived a few moments later to sweep me into his office. What he is doing for his patients today he terms as two specific treatments.

1. Ribonucleic Acid (RNA), and Deoxyribonucleic Acid (DNA), on which the RNA depends for its composition, are used to revitalise the system.

2. Serotherapy – using antibodies in the form of a serum obtained from animals which have been injected with the appropriate cells corresponding to those requiring treatment in the patient.

The RNA and DNA theory sounds complicated but is fairly simple to follow. Very basically it is explained thus: it has been proved that in every tissue there are highly specific, structurally different ribonucleic acids (RNA) which control the synthesis of the organ's or tissue's proteins – RNA of the liver, for example, allows only the formation of liver protein and those of the heart, heart protein.

In regeneration it is known that all tissue proteins must be replaced by new ones every six months, therefore the RNA is vital to that growth.

Whereas in basic cell therapy the whole cell is implanted into the patient, in this system, which was developed by well known German Professor H. Dyckerhoff in Cologne under the name of Regeneresen, only the RNA which is present in the nucleus of all cells or embryonic tissue and is essential to growth of new cells, is injected.

The RNA injections ensure that the reproduction of new cells, as described in the process of basic cell therapy, reaches peak efficiency again.

Stephan talks in staccato tones, catapaulting the words out, anxious for you to understand his beliefs and his desire to prove his methods to science. Today, he says, everyone is talking about youth. It's a new cult.

"I think it is partly our life style. People now have the ability to get far more out of life in a material sense. They travel much more than they did. There is a freedom among people that was never there before. We do not accept any more that by the time you get to so-called middle age you just forget it all, lock yourself in a back room and wait to grow old. Now people want to live their lives to the absolute limit, to the full.

"Medicine has gone through all sorts of dark ages. We have gone through the situation where if you have got a pain you take a suppressant; if you can't sleep you take a sleeping pill; if you can't get up in the morning you take a pill or two; if you are depressed you take an anti-depressant and so it goes on. But the body is such an intricate mechanism it cannot go on like that. It's so much better that we have thorough regular check-ups, that we look into any weak spots in the body and we treat it with the methods available to us today."

People come to Peter Stephan with all sorts of problems apart from the overriding one of wanting to look and feel younger or worry over the menopause, frigidity or impotency. Dr Stephan has special treatments for sexual problems. But, in addition, people come with arthritis, digestive complaints, anxiety situations and blood pressure problems.

Says Stephan: "Let's face it. They are sick to death of seeing their local doctor who does absolutely nothing else but write out a prescription."

One of the greatest criticisms levelled at Stephan by his contemporaries in the medical profession is that he is not qualified medically. He has an M.D. in homeopathic medicine. But in his defence, he says that the most important factor in getting successful cell therapy treatment is for people to go to a practitioner who knows what he or she is doing; someone who has experience in this particular treatment and is qualified to give it to them.

Certainly many G.P.'s I have spoken to completely disregard cell therapy because they know nothing about it.

Discussing its merits with one of America's leading cancer specialists and one of the most highly qualified medical men in the U.S.A., I picked him up when he poured cold water over the idea of cell therapy having any merit. To his credit he listened to me for a few moments and then said, "I withdraw those comments then. I don't know enough about it . . ." If only there were more like that.

In so many cases people read or hear about cell therapy, then go to their own doctor and ask him whether they should have it and what he thinks. He hasn't, of course, the faintest idea. He simply, therefore, gives a medical opinion which usually, being conventional, is that there is no proven merit in it.

The whole concept of body servicing is simply that – to service the body. It begins with a detailed medical examination to find out the root cause of any symptoms or conditions suffered by the patient. A sample of urine is sent to Germany for the specific, highly analytical Abderhalden test to sum up the physical condition of the patient. Blood tests are also carried out.

Any problems such as sexual hang-ups are discussed carefully and frankly. After all this, and only when tests are completed, are the specific injections of serum or RNA decided upon to correspond to organs or tissues that need treatment. If the patient is only coming for a general revitalisation course to look more youthful and healthier then a two week course of injections is prescribed.

In many cases treatment is by a course of tissue-specific antisera self-administered by the patient by means of suppositions, or these may be used as a follow-up to injection treatment.

Patients who have had cell treatment from Stephan report they generally feel happier, more relaxed and able to cope with life. Gradually they find aches and pains disappear, they have more energy than ever before and best of all they begin to look younger.

Here are some case histories that I think you will find interesting.

Sheila Black, a financial journalist now with the *Times* of London, who was treated in 1971, said that afterwards she met a well-known actress who asked her "Christ, have you had your face lifted or something?"

Another patient, a sixty-three year old writer on sexology, Robert Chartham says, "I can't understand why it happens or how it happens. All I know is that it happened to me. I had this treatment two years ago. For fifteen years before that I was crippled with osteoarthritis. In really bad winter months I was able to get about only on all fours. Within a few months of the treatment I was getting no pain, not a twinge. Now I swim half a mile a day."

A four times married, 54-year-old London columnist, James Pettigrew, had the treatment two years ago and said even his doctor agreed afterwards that he was a fitter chap.

At the end of the first month an extraordinary change in his metabolism became obvious. "For the first time in four or five years I began to feel the need of physical sex – not just once in a blue moon but almost every second day. Suddenly," he says, "I was turned on again. I felt like a young wolf in old ram's clothing. It was no mere fantasy."

In addition, he says, he began to sleep better, eat better and feel a lessening of tension. Disc and bronchitis problems from which he had been suffering cleared up and life became daily more cheerful.

He concluded: "I do know, beyond doubt, that I feel a handful of years less old than I did."

Patrick Macnee, 56-year-old star of the British T.V. *Avengers* series took the Stephan treatment and wrote: "I can now play tennis twice a day which I couldn't before. My blood pressure is normal. Many friends in my age group have died of heart attacks this year or last – I could go through an enormous list of names. Dr Stephan told me his treatment was rather like vaccinating against old age. You prevent – you don't wait for it to happen. I've got the sorest backside in the world, but the injections make me feel twenty years younger!"

People have always been quick to accuse the rejuvenators of quackery. Few know more about this sordid side of youth medicine than Peter Stephan. Since his childhood he has experienced it first hand.

He speaks of his experiences coldly and dispassionately for a man who normally bubbles with warmth.

"When my father first started cell therapy in Britain over twenty years ago, about 1952, there was tremendous criticism. They called him a quack, they called him just everything possible to call somebody if you want to insult them.

"I remember one particular day when a patient came, had treatment and that evening the police arrived at my father's clinic and said they wished to question him on a matter of fraud. They told him they had been led to believe that he had been injecting distilled water into people and saying it was something else. The funny thing was that he was just doing the accounts from Germany. They were spread across his desk. Handing a document to the police he said: 'If it's distilled water, don't you think its somewhat expensive?' The police apologised. That was only one instance."

In another, Stephan's father was involved in an action in the British Courts for calling himself "Doctor".

"My father had qualified under a different name than the one he was using. It was for personal reasons, no criminal reason at all, but he simply didn't want to practice under the family name. There was an action against him and in private chambers the judge talked to my father. He came back into Court and in his summing up said he was satisfied that the man, if not the name, was in fact qualified.

"I remember when I was very young one headline: 'Call Me Mister Says Rogue Doctor'. There were lots of things like this which you know were pretty unpleasant for him."

Stephan's father studied with Niehans and was in fact a close friend of the rejuvenator. They had great mutual respect. When Niehans visited London he never met the press, but always came quietly and always met with his old friend.

Recalls Stephan: "My father was one of the old school. He believed very strongly in what he was doing and was very genuine in his actions. He helped a large number of people. Therefore he couldn't understand why, if the press were coming to see him about something in which he was totally genuine, they should criticise him. So he allowed himself to be photographed with big syringes and all kinds of things which nowadays would be all right but twenty years ago was disastrous with those foot-in-the-door style journalists of the day looking for exposés. Too often he was alone with them instead of having a witness to back up what he said and it was their word against his.

"In my opinion my father was a very great man. He was like Niehans in that he thought what he said was quite enough. He didn't believe he had to go to great lengths and waste valuable time explaining his theories. He would simply say, 'This is the treatment, this is what it's going to do. Come, lie down and I'll give it to you.' That was all right for people with a great deal of faith but unfortunately it was quite the wrong approach in many ways.

"I was fifteen when I first saw Niehans. I was with my father and was ordered out of the clinic. I was much too young, he said, to be there and I wasn't allowed to see or do anything. Niehans' clinic was run on extremely stringent terms. It was very, very difficult for anybody to get in. Today it's open house – providing you have the right entrée card."

Was Niehans as autocratic as everybody says?

"Yes. A brilliant man, brilliant intuition, incredible foresight, incredible courage – just as Christian Barnard showed incredible courage with the first heart transplant. But a lot of people cannot understand it when a man takes his training and puts it to use rather than just staying within the routine. They think there is something wrong. It has always amazed me that when a man who spends that amount of time learning the profession, learning about the body and may spend years in practice – never does anything on his own, never steps out of the normal routine."

Stephan didn't meet his father until he was thirteen-years-old. He was brought up by his mother in Yorkshire. At their first meeting they were not even introduced as father and son. An uncle, on the pretext that he needed treatment, took his nephew along with him to the doctor.

Recalls Stephan now: "He sat and talked to me and asked me all sorts of questions. I couldn't understand why he was asking me what I was going to do with my future, whether I was going to study or go and dig holes in the road. But it's a funny thing between people – I liked him immediately and I warmed towards him although I didn't have the faintest notion of who he was at all. I mean, one hears these stories of how you look your parents in the eye and you know it's your father. I didn't."

Later, Stephan's father invited him to London and they spent a lot of time talking. Finally it was decided that young Stephan would follow in his father's footsteps and join the practice.

"I was fascinated with what was going on. To me it was absolute sense that if a part of the body is not functioning then you should treat that part naturally. To stuff yourself with antibiotics and antidepressants was absolutely crazy. And I saw the result. I saw patients come in, and a number of them I saw carried in and I saw them three months later. I saw women patients who you literally did not recognise after treatment, the change was so dramatic.

"We used to have long discussions my father and I. When we met we went through a great loving phase, then we went through a great hate phase, and then fortunately in the latter part of his life, thank God, we went through another loving phase when we were great together. We travelled around the world together, we were more like brothers than anything else.

"He was only sixty-two when he died – he had a horrible death, he was in pain for almost six years. He had spent six years in an internment camp during the War and suffered as a result of that. The day before he died he was still treating patients and the man was in such pain he couldn't stand, he couldn't lie, couldn't sit. When he died in 1965 I closed the practice for that year."

In those days, Stephan recalled, people were much more secretive about youth treatments. "We used to have sometimes a husband and wife who would come at the same time and neither knew the other was there. Really, I'm not joking. And they used to go home and stay in bed and pretend they had the 'flu.' "

It was also a period when many quacks climbed onto the lucrative cell therapy bandwaggon. Stephan speaks of them bitterly: "There was a policeman and an osteopath who got together in Canada, got into a car one day, drove to a farm, picked up a sheep, took it home, dissected it and injected it into their patients. The patients died of gasgangrene, of course. I almost sent a lawyer across to fight it. Not for them, I couldn't care less about them frankly. But the fact that they claimed this was Niehans' cell therapy – and it was not.

"Then I had a friend who telephoned me to say an Australian was advertising cell therapy in this country. The friend came over and showed me this ad and there was a whole list of treatments said to be cell therapy in capsule form. So I rang this man using another name saying I was interested. To cut a long story short he told me he knew Peter Stephan very well and had met his father. I pretended I was meeting Stephan for a drink at six o'clock and I would get him to telephone.

"Well, I couldn't wait for six o'clock to come. It turned out the man had been buying placenta from Mexico, putting it into capsules and selling it to people as cell therapy. The reason he had met my father was when he tried to sell him some of the placenta and my father sent him packing. On his way out he had happened to pass me in the hallway which was why he claimed to 'know' me. I told him I had been in touch with Niehans and was going to take legal action. The man went back to Australia.

"Every year you hear of something else. They do a quick rake off and then stop . . ."

Stephan issues a serious warning to would-be cell therapy patients. Watch out for over-charging.

One doctor close to his own surgery charges $3600/£1800, sometimes more. "Some people are charging crazy amounts, unbelievable. We have enormous expenses here, we are very serious about financing our research and are giving grants to research in London, America, Switzerland and Germany but we still don't charge thousands of pounds."

One well known cell therapist, according to Stephan, travels around Europe regularly choosing one patient a year. He waits until he finds a suitable, fat-pocketed industrialist, meets him socially, sends flowers to his wife, treats him and then charges a fantastic fee.

However, Stephan says, "I'm much happier about the way things in this business are going now than I have been in the past. You see one of the greatest problems with this so called youth situation is that everybody tries to get in on the bandwagon and they do. We have all kinds of people giving all kinds of things – the hair transplant business for example at the moment is crazy. I want to ensure first of all for the benefit of the patient that the sort of treatment they are getting has been proven to work, that it is efficient and that they are not going to be taken to the cleaners for it."

Stephan's comments only serve to underline what has gone so far in this book – that there are countless millions of people today who are ill, dissatisfied with themselves and the way they look and who just don't have the capacity to do what they want to in life. Until the day comes when one panacea, one remedy for all these ills, a youth treatment without equal is discovered – and it may be just around the corner – then I cannot stress strongly enough the need for caution to avoid those quacks and charlatans.

Stephan's fees vary between $1000/£500 and $1200/£600 for the full course of treatment. His address is:

The Harley Place Private Clinic Ltd.,
27, Harley Place,
Harley Street,
London W.1.

CHAPTER ELEVEN

Romania's Fountain Of Youth

"I am convinced that people can live longer, remain healthier and die with more dignity than they do now."

Professor Dr Ana Aslan M.D.
Director of the Romanian Institute
of Gerontology and Geriatrics

An avenue of majestic horse-chestnuts within an old walled garden, tumbling with dusty lilacs and the dark red roses which abound everywhere in Bucharest, leads the way to Romania's Fountain of Youth presided over by the world famous Professor Dr Ana Aslan.

For nearly thirty years the Romanian Institute of Gerontology and Geriatrics, of which she is the Director, has been a Mecca to thousands of pilgrims seeking the wonder treatment which Dr Aslan claims can hold off old age.

Dr Aslan is 82, a small, bouncy, brown-haired ball of energy, and is easily the best known youth doctor alive in the world today. And if she is telling the truth she is also a pretty good advertisement for her own treatment which she claims she has been taking for well over 20 years.

Her therapy has been and still is sought by an impressive array of Royals, Presidents and showbiz stars. Aslan refuses to reveal her patients' identities but it is persistently repeated that they have included Nikita Kruschev, Sukarano of Indonesia, Charles de Gaulle, King Saud of Saudi Arabia, Ghanian president, Dr Nkrumah, Kirk Douglas and Lilian Gish.

After cellular therapy, of which we have talked, Dr Aslan's Procaine based revitalisation drug, Gerovital H3, is probably the most widely talked about youth treatment anywhere in the world among those, even mildly, intrigued by the idea of staying young.

According to Aslan, who travels thousands of miles each year bombarding scientific meetings with her theories, her treatment can increase the average person's life span by up to 15 years. It can also, she confidently says, cure conditions such as baldness, grey hair, fading vision, deafness, wrinkling, skin troubles like psoriasis and the most common male problem, impotence, as well as showing good results in such a variety of cases as arthritis, arteriosclerosis, high blood pressure, Parkinson's Disease, angina pectoris and post myocardium infarct.

If Dr Aslan is to be believed her treatment is certainly worthy of world-wide medical attention, and many doctors have slowly but surely been won over to support her cause and, indeed, to use her treatment on their own patients.

Predictably, however, like all youth drugs, Gerovital is still a subject of world wide medical controversy. Its effects and results have been examined and fiercely argued by medical sceptics at numerous international conferences and symposiums specially set up for the purpose since it was discovered by Aslan 30 years ago.

Nevertheless, despite the continuing medical battle or perhaps because of it, as more and more doctors agree Gerovital has some merits, 20,000 patients pour into Romania every year to receive the injections or as Aslan calls it take her "cure".

They come in the main from Britain, Spain, Italy, Singapore, France, Holland, Germany, Sweden and the U.S. Many more people around the world, many of them doctors, their wives and families, have the jabs from their own G.P.s. The drug is available in 73 countries made under licence, according to the Aslan formula, or in similar versions such as KH3, also made from a Procaine base, from Britain to Australia and as far afield as Japan.

Aslan argues that KH3 and similar copies are not the same as her formula. The manufacturers of KH3, Schwarzhaupt, with headquarters in Cologne, West Germany, tell me it is identical, and tests being carried out by a number of eminent scientists are, in fact, based on double blind tests using KH3. In some countries the Procaine treatment, available in injection and pill forms, is sold only on doctors' prescriptions but in others, such as Britain and Germany, it is freely available over the chemists' counters.

However, a word of warning for anyone thinking of embarking. First of all, patients in the Aslan Clinic and elsewhere undergo a complete series of medical tests before treatment and, in addition, one in every five thousand may have allergic reactions to Procaine. Secondly, unlike cell therapy, Gerovital treatment is no one-off affair. It means repeated injections and pill treatments continuing over the years or, admits Aslan, the effects will simply fade and you will be back to square one.

Following in the wake of the summer surge of American jet package holidaymakers who go to Romania on a two week "get young" visit before heading off to "do" Europe, I went to Bucharest to find out about Aslan and Gerovital treatment for myself. Not this time, however, to have the treatment myself but to meet and talk to those who had. It was a fascinating journey.

Ana Aslan is regarded in Romania today as something in the nature of a national heroine. The people reserve for her the sort of adulation usually accorded to football stars or, at the least, Olympic gymnasts – certainly not what one would imagine for an elderly woman scientist dabbling in the realms of science fiction against the down-to-earth rigid and rather humourless background of modern day Romania.

The mere mention of her name at the airport as I went through immigration and currency checks brought out the smiles among the grim faced military officials.

"Dr Aslan? – Of course, of course – " as I replied to their queries about the purpose of my visit.

They waved me through as if it was inconceivable that I could have come for any other reason.

"But you are too young," one of them said with a hint of the old romantic Romania of the past, bowing flatteringly.

I didn't bother to explain I hadn't come to have the cure – but to hear about it. After all, why should they have cared, anyway? One tourist's dollars are much the same as another's in the poor-relation Romanian tourist industry's wide open coffers, an industry which blatantly advertises their keep young holidays as Romania's Fountain of Youth.

Aslan has not always been regarded by her countrymen with such respect. Even today she is not so warmly regarded by some of her colleagues in the medical profession. She has many times had to run the gauntlet of accusations from her political masters that she was a charlatan, a liar and a cheat – even though she has always had support in some pretty high quarters.

Despite the fact that her drug was offically licenced in Romania in 1957 she has many times come under fire from the Romanian Communist Party for what they claimed were "false theories". They even publicly described her clinic as a "phoney Fountain of Youth" as they tried in vain to discredit her work, accusing her of sheltering reactionaries and former landowners in her clinic. Even, on occasions, her passport was withdrawn.

Nevertheless, the plucky, bouncy, little Professor carried on undaunted; experimenting, testing, documenting her results with painstaking and unflagging care as she gathered her evidence of the successes of her treatment and began to publish the results.

Aslan first realised the potential of Procaine in 1949. Many claims that Procaine therapy had a stimulating effect on the central nervous system had been made since 1930. As it happened Aslan had not read them, a fact which was later to lead to embarrassment when she published her first paper and was accused of plagiarism.

However, at the time she was pursuing her own theories, and when a young medical student at the Imisoara Faculty of Medicine in Transylvania was suffering with his knee totally locked from arthritis and was in severe pain, Dr Aslan asked if he would volunteer for Procaine treatment. She injected a large dose of Procaine direct into the artery of his leg and to the surprise of the youth and indeed to Aslan's amazement the pain vanished and the patient found he could almost immediately bend his leg. Within days he left the hospital – cured.

Following this success, Aslan continued to experiment but decided to use a more acid Procaine solution – the first Gerovital. It is based, as I have described, on Procaine, the drug better known under its brand name of Novacaine, widely used by dentists as an anaesthetic. Today, Aslan's solution also contains benzoic acid and potassium metadisulphite to stabilise the drug and induce changes in the Procaine's activity.

There followed between 1949 and 1951 a series of tests on young and old patients, during which Aslan concluded that the Gerovital H3, besides its local action, exerted a general action on both the central nervous system level and on other tissues.

Her critics, among the strongest being doctors in the United States where the Food and Drug Administration only allowed tests to begin as late as 1973, said that the results of Gerovital were purely psychological.

Aslan's claims were much more positive and far more dramatic. While agreeing that her drug does have anti-depressant qualities resulting in people generally feeling better, she says firmly that it also has much more far reaching effects. "It slows the rate of ageing, reverses premature ageing and ameliorates old age diseases," she says.

In all her early efforts Dr Aslan was backed by the powerful Professor C.I. Parhon, himself a noted physician and investigator into the ageing process. More importantly, as far as Aslan was concerned, when King Michael of Romania abdicated in 1948, Parhon, of whom she had been a student, became first President of the new Romanian Peoples' Republic.

It was fairly predictable that three years later, when he set up an institute for the study of diseases and causes of ageing, he should place his brilliant former pupil, Ana Aslan, in charge of it. It was the first Gerontology Centre of its kind in the world and there experiments into the Procaine therapy were able to begin in earnest, not the least of its advantages being a permanent supply of elderly patients on which to try it.

During the next ten years Dr Aslan treated more than 10,000 patients, carefully documenting medical results. Clinical and experimental tests were carried out not only on humans but also on rats, birds and even micro-organisms. With centres opening throughout the country under her control, Aslan was able to turn Romania into a sort of national test bed for her treatment.

"Our purpose," she says, "was not just to treat old people but to investigate the ideas of Parhon that ageing is a pathologic dystrophic phenomenon that can be modified by therapeutic intervention with enzymes, hormones or vitamins. With his help I separated the patients into three groups, each to receive a different treatment – Vitamin E, Extract of Pineal Gland or Procaine. We had a control group but it was not treated with placebo, only symptomatically."

After three years they examined results from physiology, intelligence tests and patient reactions and found that the best results were being obtained in the Procaine group.

The results were astonishing. Patients who could scarcely walk due to the crippling effects of arthritis found their muscles had loosened up and they could move easily again, the pain gone. Sufferers from high blood pressure found their condition normalised and the pain of angina pectoris caused by clogged arteries to the heart, diminished.

Improvements were found in memory and concentration – one of the most feared hazards of old age; liver spots or blotches of pigmentation, one of the most tell-tale signs of senility, either faded or disappeared. Nails were found to improve and thick, chalky toenails so common in the elderly were smooth and pink again. Skin regained its elasticity and in some cases patients found their grey hair regained its natural colour or, in cases of balding, new hair grew again.

Other illnesses connected with the ageing syndrome, which Dr Aslan says she has found can be improved, are: diseases of the central nervous system such as Parkinson's disease, spasms, thrombosis, haemorrhage, muscular contractions or paralysis; disturbances affecting men's and women's sexual climax; generalised arteriosclerosis or conditions such as coronary, cerebral or peripheric arteriosclerosis, or the conditions post myocardium infarct; chronic rheumatism or orthopaedic diseases accompanied by osteoporosis, post fracture sequelae, etc; chronic bronchitis; ulcer diseases such as gastro duodenal ulcer.

The treatment also claims to be able to improve deafness and fading vision as well as generally improving both physical and mental capacity.

Could it really be that here was a valuable tool in the fight to control the ageing process? Aslan has believed from the start that it is . . .

Let us look at exactly what the treatment involves. Patients from overseas normally go through a two-week treatment course involving a full medical and then twelve injections of Gerovital H3, one per day, followed by a ten day rest period and then two pills a day for another twelve days. The pills, of course, can be taken home. The medical, X-rays, cardiograph, etc., are to determine the best course of treatment for the patient's individual condition, if it is being undertaken for reasons other than rejuvenation.

Today, visitors can, if they choose, have treatment at Aslan's headquarters, the Institute of Gerontology and Geriatrics in Minastirea Caldarusani Street where Dr Aslan, with her right hand Executive Director Dr Alexander Ciuca, stage manages the Gerovital story for world wide consumption.

There, striped pyjama clad oldsters sit or wander in the flower scented grounds. But it is an old grey stone building, colourless and rather forbidding and despite the gleaming modern laboratories, which are Aslan's pride and joy, I found the institutionalised atmosphere, like that of so many old peoples' homes, depressing. That is why I assume the majority of Romania's youth visitors choose to have their treatment at any one of a number of modern hotels and sanatoria scattered around the capital, coastal and mountain regions where they can combine treatment with pleasure.

I visited several in the city and country and found them relaxing and pleasant and quite unlike the usual clinics in either aspect or atmosphere. For example, the Otopeni Clinic, 18 kilometres from the centre of Bucharest and conveniently near the airport is like an old hunting lodge. The approach through high gates is up a long winding tree-lined drive with private woodlands on each side.

The pillared front entrance is reached by a broad gravel sweep. The main part of the hotel is approached by an impressive long marble gallery with red carpet and scattered green chairs leading to wide airy corridors. The bedrooms I saw were also large, more like private sitting-rooms with gracious sofas where visitors can relax in the afternoon after treatment. The windows lead to private balconies, each overlooking the expansive gardens, rather like a mini Versailles. Below is a pleasant heated indoor swimming pool, tourists and handicraft shops and a conference hall and a gracious old library with volumes in all languages. In addition, the sanitorium has medical consulting rooms, laboratories, X-ray and electro-cardiography rooms, electro-therapy, hydro-therapy and recovery rooms as well as massage facilities and a medical gymnasium.

There are only 40 rooms and the clinic preserves its peaceful, old world atmosphere by taking a maximum of 80 patients. The cost is from $940/£469 for two weeks which includes flight, room, full board and treatment, or from $1255/£628 for three weeks.

To those who prefer independence it is possible to have treatment while staying in a private villa on the shores of the Snagov Lake. Alternatively, there are several modern hotels with all the facilities the most energetic keep-fit guest could require.

The 500 bed Parc Hotel which I visited in Bucharest, for example, has a superb gymnasium for special slimming gymnastics, Olympic-style indoor pool, sauna and turkish baths, vibratory and hand massage, and bowling, golf, mini-golf and tennis facilities. In addition, in the first floor medical block there are six medical consulting rooms, a laboratory, X-ray rooms and electro-therapy sections. Special exercises under supervision are laid on for those with backbone infections, respiratory troubles, children with various ailments, or simply for those who need slimming and generally toning up, just like a normal health farm holiday.

A new similar centre has recently opened at the Flora Cure Hotel on the outskirts of Bucharest.

At what age do patients come for treatment? That, says Aslan, is the thousand dollar question. Many patients come for treatment between the ages of 40 and 45. No, it's not too early so don't be surprised. Aslan recommends patients to start at 40 as a preventative measure before the signs of old age can get a hold. The majority of visitors, however, are between 60 and 70 years old.

At the Parc Hotel I was told that patients usually return for treatment every two years but in Europe, where travel is easy and cheap, they often return for a booster each year.

The main centres for treatment are:

In Bucharest and its surroundings – the Flora Cure Hotel, Otopeni Sanatorium and the Cure Centre at Snagov.

In the more picturesque climate resorts there are spas at:

Felix, Herculaene, Caciulata-Calimanesti, and at Eforie Nord and Neptun on the Romanian Black Sea coast, all of which have supervised branches of the National Gerontology and Geriatric Institute under Dr Aslan.

Enquiries should be made through branches of the Romanian National Tourist office or the Carpati-Bucharest National Tourist Office.

Many hospitals have now tried tests on the treatment but, obviously, to print them all would be long, involved and tedious for the layman. Most reports are freely available.

For example, a test carried out in the first internal hospital of the Medical Faculty of Sarajevo using KH3 Geriatricum-Schwarzhaupt was tried on fifty patients aged between forty-four and eighty-four, including thirty-eight men and twelve women all in hospital.

Summarising, and I quote: "We can say that the product exercised a generally invigorating effect producing a favourable influence especially on diseases of old age; this we found in the case of 70% of our test personnel. It seems, too, that the product has a certain anabolic action, and this is manifest by an improvement in the serum proteins, particularly the albumin's, and by an improvement in the protein level. The digestion of our old patients is favourably influenced by KH3. In like manner KH3 also displayed a stimulating effect on the blood picture, meaning on the erythropoiesis.

"When it was a question of symptoms within the scope of the central nervous system and also when it was a question of cerebral sclerosis and dementia senilis, good therapeutic results were obtained with KH3. The sensorium brightened up in the case of more than half of our test persons and insomnia was improved (29). Headaches were reduced in a number of cases (17).

"All test persons tolerated the product excellently. One of the most interesting results, taken from a number of doctors publishing test papers, was the improvement in memory retention and mental mobility in old people after treatment."

In addition, I spoke to a large number of doctors and their wives or patients using KH3 on a regular basis. All described higher energy, smoother skin and one man rang me to say he had been bald but now had a full head of hair!

A doctor's wife who had suffered seriously with arteriosclerosis said she was much improved and could get about with relative ease. All reported feeling fitter and in better health while on the pills than they were without them. All the people I spoke to were in the fifty to seventy years age bracket.

CHAPTER TWELVE

Pills Over The Counter

"It is quite useless for people who wish to keep young and active to drug themselves with sedatives, tranquillisers and sleeping pills."
Barbara Carland, novelist

It is all very well discussing the amazing health and rejuvenation clinics dotted round the world but what – if anything – is available for you and I over the chemist's counter at home – or even on prescription from a sympathetic local doctor?

Not all of us, after all, can jet around the world in pursuit of youth. Many more of us, with financial and family ties to consider, are only able to try any remedy on offer to help us keep young in the privacy of our own homes. That applies even more so if we have a sceptical or unsympathetic partner likely to ridicule our attempts as vain or stupid. But let them keep their old-fashioned views – our beliefs and the fun of discovery can be our own.

The choice varies from country to country depending on the particular stringency of Government health and drug laws, but as increasing numbers of natural health food shops open and as the demand for vitality and rejuvenation treatments expands, too, slowly but surely more products are becoming available.

In the last two years many new youth/health treatments – most of them carefully labelled as diet, vitamin supplements or slimming products – have mushroomed on to the market to be snapped up by customers-in-the-know.

As Roland Steinbach of the giant Schwarzhaupt Drug Company in Cologne, West Germany, told me: "The stress of life is so great today, particularly for people over 50, they are looking for drugs and vitamins that will give vitality, improve health and reduce depression."

I have searched chemists' counters on my route across the world sifting, buying, talking and trying to find out which among the staggering array are value for money. Clearly every week there are new products making new claims and it is impossible to mention them all. I am, therefore, listing only those which have a long record of success or where there is sufficient medical evidence in their favour to make it worthwhile exploring the possibilities for yourself.

KH3

Based on Doctor Aslan's Romanian formula, Gerovital H3, KH3 is one of the most commonly available treatments in pill form over the counter. However, beware of the many variations – and there are quite a number on the market.

Dr Steinbach's firm, Schwarzhaupt, have been manufacturing KH3 – oral Procaine-Hematoporphyrine since 1959. It was the first youth drug of its kind in the field and today they corner 40% of the market in Germany alone. Germany, of course, is way ahead in its view of youth treatments. Most chemists there stock a wide selection of youth and health treatments, and rejuvenation as a medical field is no longer regarded with suspicion, but accepted as a sensible and necessary part of modern-day preventative medicine.

American tourists have long been raiding German health stores to smuggle home supplies for themselves and friends, since it is banned in their own country. U.K. physicians have traditionally been just as firmly against such treatments, pooh-poohing them in general as so much quackery and nonsense and it is only now beginning to gradually change.

KH3 has long been one of the most popular and reportedly successful rejuvenation treatments, and throughout the world many thousands of people are taking KH3 daily in pill form. Many of them are doctors and their wives, to whom I have spoken. Many more doctors regularly obtain KH3, imported on prescription, for their patients in Britain and including my own G.P. in Australia.

Dr Steinbach told me his company felt that the pills give much the same effect as injections, but are so much easier to take in capsule form. It is a point on which Dr Ana Aslan does not agree. She continues to uphold her belief that there is extra benefit in her injections given in Romania, but there is no medical evidence for her theory.

Today, seventy-three countries import KH3, including Britain, Australia and Japan, most of it made in Germany, some in Cork, Eire.

Schwarzhaupt are cautious in their claims for KH3. "No, it is not a wonder pill," they say. "In the field of medicine today there are still no wonder pills. But it is certainly possible to take these pills and look better and feel better."

At the moment Schwarzhaupt are involved in long-term research plans with doctors all over Europe to prove scientifically the beneficial effects of their drug. The company say carefully that their treatment has been shown to restore hair growth in balding patients, restore hair colour and frequently improve sexual function. Patients go further by reporting a new youthfulness in the way they feel, lessening of wrinkles, new elasticity in their skin texture and improvement in many of the degenerative illnesses associated with age.

For patients aged under 55 it is recommended that one capsule a day should be taken for five months, then a break of two to three months and repeat. Older patients need one a day. Patients who have taken the treatment for between six to ten years have been shown to have no harmful side-effects.

A box of 30 capsules costs DM14.95 and a box of 90 capsules costs DM39.80. In Britain capsules are £2.48 for 30 and £10.54 for 150.

Similar versions of the KH3 treatment have been brought out by various pharmaceutical companies, cutting out the Procaine content to comply with local drug laws and enable it to be sold openly without prescription – as a vitamin. One variant in Australia was TH3 now being sold as JH3. When it first came on the market hundreds of youth seekers queued clamouring for it overnight at one chemist's shop.

In Britain other similar pills on the market, selling as H3 Factor supplements are: Multivitamin/Mineral Plus H3 (80 tablets $3/£1.50); Maxivits with H3 (20 tablets $3/£1.50) and Minivits with H3 (50 tablets $3/£1.50) and Celaton CH3 Tri-Plus (120 tablets $10/£5.02).

Municaps

This is another youth pill on the open market, recommended as a type of KH3 but with a quicker energy and health boost for the under-45's.

Launched in Germany in January 1976, the pills were available to anyone over the chemist's counter – and had an instant success as a best-seller. Taken after a cup of coffee it makes you feel instantly refreshed and clearer in the brain – particularly after a hangover!

A box of 30 capsules costs DM19.90 ($10/£5) and one of 90 ampules DM48.50 ($25/£12.50).

The pills contain Vitamins B-1, B-2, B-6 and B-12 plus Nicotinoyl Procaine and it was first developed in Austria.

It is recommended to improve cell respiration and utilisation of oxygen by the cells. It has a positive effect on metabolism of protein, carbohydrate and fat, lowers the level of cholesterol in the blood and, therefore, helps guard against arteriosclerosis. In addition, it is claimed to be an agent in regulating blood pressure, enhancing physical and intellectual efficiency and, therefore, overall potency.

Among its effects are said to be an improvement of poor memory, a raised performance in sporting demands, improvement where there is shortness of breath on walking or climbing stairs, less fatigue from physical work or muscle pains on strenuous activity.

It is also said to help in mental relaxation, in daily work stress, in the home, fear of examinations or severe mental strain.

It can relieve restlessness and sleep disturbances such as nervous difficulty in falling asleep, tension on awakening in the morning, stomach upsets caused by nerves and nerve stress resulting in increased intake of alcohol and cigarettes.

Ginseng

The latest and most popular rejuvenation buy over the counter is a Chinese remedy almost as old as the mystic East itself – Ginseng. Grown mainly in remote parts of China, Korea and Siberia, this highly prized root plant has a history dating back over 5000 years.

It is said to have been a highly regarded wonder cure for many diseases in China and Tibet as early as 3000 B.C. as well as an aid to longevity and an aphrodisiac.

Today its life-giving properties and its value as an anti-stress agent and tonic are becoming equally widely known in the West, as it was to the noblemen of the ancient Orient, and it is a best-seller in health food shops from Los Angeles to Australia and back to the wilds of the North of England.

Demand far exceeds supply as the precious plant which grows from seed is not ready for harvest until six years after planting. It can be seen, therefore, that the cost and risks involved in its production are enormous.

The stories and legends surrounding Ginseng's health-giving powers are legion, and from its earliest days of the third century the root, which takes the shape of a man, (its Chinese name "Jin Seng" means "Man Plant") is said to have possessed divine power. Stories of its wonder cures have been written and passed down through the centuries and every Chinese family swears by its health and youth-giving qualities, although they are often loath to talk to strangers about them.

Today the original Ginseng root – Panax Ginseng – is grown as part of a national policy in both China and Korea, the Korean variety being accepted as the most potent available giving superior strength. But it is closely rivalled by Siberian Ginseng, the Eleutheron Ginseng – from the similar plant family, Eleutherococcus Senticus. The Russian variety is said to have been planted in the Siberian mountains from seed obtained in Korea during the war of 1950-53. Whatever the origin, this Siberian Ginseng is now highly regarded by Soviet scientists for its health-giving powers. At present, research is still being carried out in Russia, France, Britain and America to try to find out more about its mystical properties.

Because potential varies between plants of different origins, besides the genuine Korean and Chinese roots other varieties have sprung up in America, India and Japan, it has therefore been difficult for scientists to draw definite conclusions.

In the East, Orientals have always regarded Ginseng as a source of long life as well as an aphrodisiac. Modern scientists also believe Ginseng is a means of delaying the signs of ageing and experiments have shown that with laboratory animals Ginseng even reversed the ageing process. Its specific value in relation to disease is as yet unsubstantiated, but there is no question as to its value for thousands of people as a tonic and anti-stress and fatigue factor.

Most Westeners, of course, buy their Ginseng in preparation packets often combined with vitamins, although many real health addicts prefer to chew the root as did the Orientals. Here, however, for the do–it–yourself health fiend is the original health drink recipe direct from an old Chinese friend: the resulting liquid is recommended as an ideal remedy for any circulatory and metabolism malfunction which means, say the Chinese, just about anything, as well as keeping you looking young and preventing hair turning grey.

Take a glass bottle with largish opening. Cut 100g dry Ginseng into small pieces (you can obtain this from a friendly health food shop if you order it well in advance). Put the pieces in the bottle together with 100 cc of spirit of Japanese rice wine (Saké), available from Japanese supermarkets, some wine shops and delicatessens. Place the lid on the bottle. It takes about three weeks for the extract of Ginseng to blend into the alcohol. Drink one or two small 10 cc cupfuls about twice a day. When the liquor has been consumed you can use the remainder of the Ginseng root by adding to chicken soup with a little salt. As an alternative you can add sliced root ginger into the original mixture.

The combinations of Ginseng plus vitamins available over the counter are enormous, and indeed it is important to watch out for imitations as some of the inferior Ginseng on the market is being sold to look like the original Korean variety – so read the labels carefully.

Most popular versions being sold in Britain and America are combined with vitamins such as B-6 and E and B-15.

Prices vary enormously. To give you a few examples: you can buy original Korean extract 600mg for $5/£2.75, 32 capsules combined with B-6 and E, 60 tablets for $5/£2.50, and Siberian Ginseng 600mg, 30 capsules, for $6/£2.99. An intriguing formula which is proving popular also is Vitamin F and E together with Chinese Ginseng 250mg and Zinc, 25 tablets $4/£2.

F-500

This is one of the latest, most exciting over-the-counter discoveries. For years, vitamin E was the fashionable vitamin on the international health scene. Now Vitamin F looks like making a name for itself.

Authoress Barbara Cartland, herself a glamorous advertisement for healthy advancing years – whisper it quietly, she is 77 – says she has made an amazing discovery. After using F-500 containing an elusive new vitamin factor, Miss Cartland says:

"Here at last, in my opinion, is a real source of youth for those who wish for it. Since I have been taking F-500 I have found that not only do I feel extremely well but my brain is more active. I have also discovered that a face cream which contains Vitamin FF has had a spectacular effect on the appearance and texture of my skin."

So what is this miracle youth pill which gets such a glowing report from the Queen of romantic novelists, who still writes every day of her life, runs a large house, entertains lavishly, travels and has a wide and active social life?

Ever since 1953 it has been known that a number of bodily disorders stemmed from a dificiency of Vitamin F. Ordinary 9 : 12 Vitamin F (Linoleic Acid) has long been advocated for treating degenerative disorders such as heart disease, acne, ulcers and skin disorders.

To cater for the demand, polyunsaturated vegetable oils containing Vitamin F, such as Safflower and Sunflower oils, have become popular. But it was discovered that within the body ordinary Vitamin F was converted into a far more valuable 6 : 9 : 12 Vitamin F (Octadecatrienoic Acid).

Recently, however, a new rich, natural source of this double FF factor vitamin has been found and is being sold in health shops across Britain. It is thought that due to the stress of today's life style and the results of junk foods, sugar and pollutants that modern man may require much more of the F vitamin than ever in the past.

Its most vital function includes building body tissues and it is involved in body functions such as structural fat development, cell functions and prostaglandin production.

Now, as a result of research, chemists have found this new source of Vitamin FF and with it a whole new health potential. This 6 : 9 : 12 vitamin has been developed into F-500 gelatine capsules which contain 500 mg of natural edible oil which is made up of ordinary Vitamin F plus the super 6 : 9 : 12 Vitamin F plus other fatty acids for people over 50. For the under-40's there is a tablet FF-100 which contains less oil.

Miss Cartland reports it gives a feeling of well-being all over the body as well as a general firming of the abdomen. In addition, there is a Vitamin FF face cream which she says has a fantastic effect on the skin. She says:

"I am confident that in time it will even remove old age wrinkles. It is completely free from any form of allergy and I have found it effective, even on the delicate tops of my eye-lids to take away the crepeness. I am quite certain that if I continue with this treatment I shall find myself getting younger both in mind and body and this, after all, is what we need. I am convinced that F-500 does combine in re-creating youth both in mind and body."

The cost of F-500 capsules is 30 for $7/£3.30, 90 for $19/£9.50.
The Vitamin FF face-cream is $5/£2.30 for a 42g jar.

RNA
Ribonucleic Acids are the latest tablet diet supplement for help in memory retention, failure of which is one of the surest and earliest signs of old age.

RNA – the genetic building material – which forms with DNA (Deoxyribonucleic Acid), the basis of the living cell, comes from the very source of life. It has been shown that as we get older the body seems unable to keep up enough supplies of RNA and it is this loss that causes the general feeling of ageing and in particular memory loss.

RNA therapy is becoming more and more widely known. London's Peter Stephan is one of its leading practitioners. However, RNA is available in tablet form now – price $8/£3.90 for 45 tablets.

Royal Jelly

This is another over-the-counter treatment which has shown consistent effectiveness in countering the effects of ageing. Its considerable power in increasing energy, buoyancy, fighting depression, fatigue, sleeplessness and restoring health after illness is said to be due to the fact that Royal Jelly is the food of the Queen Bee larvae, and is secreted by young worker bees exclusively as food for young Queens-to-be. The Queen Bee is known to be almost immune to disease and she lives 30 times longer than the average worker bee.

Most people who take Royal Jelly as a regular part of their diet report fantastic results in promoting fitness and health.

Prices vary from $4.70/£2.35 for 50 Royal Jelly tablets combined with Vitamins A, D-3 and E to $3.60/£1.80 for 100g of pure Royal Jelly.

Rejuvenating Cosmetics

Every cosmetic ever to hit the lucrative beauty market claims that it – and it alone – can give a woman the natural fresh and youthful complexion she craves. Others, usually the more expensive the product the more exotic the claims, hold out hopes of vanishing wrinkles, debagged eyes, dewy skin and that eternally youthful look even when Madam is clearly well and truly past it.

But what of the products made specifically by the rejuvenators themselves? Women like Dr Aslan and men like Peter Stephan and the cell therapy men of La Prairie? And I know that hundreds of society women who have visited Aslan's clinics in Romania clamour annually to get hold of her Gerovital face-creams. Whether they work, clearly I cannot say. I can only tell you of their existence and that they are made of a similar formula to her youth cure and contain Procaine.

The Gerovital range includes cleanser, toner, night cream, moisturiser and even shampoo.

Another range which was raved over by Theodora Barbulescu at the Institute of Gerontology in Bucharest, is called Pell-Amar, and is based on the health-giving muds in the south of Romania. It is extracted from the mud springs. The products are comparatively inexpensive, unglamorously packaged, but are bought by the ton-load by American and European women tourists.

On the subject of make-up, Peter Stephan in London is on the verge of launching his own range of cosmetics. In his own words, "I have recently made two quite important breakthroughs in the subject of cosmetology using cellular extracts of skin."

The first is called Peter Stephan Complete Skin Care which will be available only from his clinic. The second is a gel – the result of enormous amounts of research to get the balance right.

He says, "Initially it was meant to be a cosmetic, but now it is totally for use in such skin ailments as acne, psoriasis, comodones and other lesions of the skin which are so often embarrassing to people."

The research work was carried out in a London hospital and laboratories in Switzerland, and Stephan reports dramatic results in all the conditions he mentions. The cream will sell for around $30/£15 and will be available from The Harley Place Swiss Clinic, 27 Harley Place, Harley Street, London W.1.

At La Prairie in Switzerland, the clinic originated by Professor Paul Niehans, they are today carrying his cell therapy treatments one step further – by applying fresh embryonic cells directly to the skin itself.

While treating burns patients in the past with their dermatological placenta gel they found that not only did it act as a healing agent but also had an excellent effect in stimulating the facial skin and smoothing wrinkles. As a result, they have launched a whole new range of cell therapy skin care products, including day and night creams, an anti-wrinkle cream and a twice weekly mask, a neck treatment and a tightening and revitalising cellular body treatment.

At present the range like the treatment is too extortionately expensive for all but the rich or perhaps desperate – $240/£120 for a set of five products. In addition the Cellular Neck Treatment costs $80/£40 and the body treatment $40/£20 – all in expensive-looking silver and white jars and bottles. They are available from the clinic in Clarens-Montreux, from Harrods in Knightsbridge, London, and Saks, Fifth Avenue, New York.

CHAPTER THIRTEEN

The Hollywood Youth Kick

"The only way to grow old gracefully is to be involved emotionally with your own body"

Vidal Sassoon

Vidal Sassoon, the world's top hairdresser and now one of Hollywood's resident beautiful people, knows what he is talking about when it comes to youth and beauty.

In terms of diet, nutrition, health foods, health farms, exercise and relaxation or any other treatments on the world scene likely to keep old age from showing, as well as adding a few years onto the life span, Vidal can claim to be an international expert. If there's half a chance it may work he's given it a go – personally.

In addition, with his ear constantly to the film world grapevine, chatting and mixing with the scores of millionaires and stars among his friends and clients, there's not much he doesn't know about what they are all getting up to in order to keep their Beautiful Plus status. The tricks and treatments they are employing with deadly seriousness in order to keep their names and faces flashing up in showbiz lights or, at the very least, in the social rat race.

Vidal at fifty-one looks a good ten years younger than his age. Nobody could deny he is a terrific advert for the youth kick. Boyish, lean and suntanned, he is the envy of most of his contemporaries as well as many much younger men, thanks to his almost fanatical attention and dedicated involvement with his body and keeping himself feeling and looking good.

When we met again, after a period of almost ten years, I could honestly say he looked scarcely a day older than the glamorous young Vidal I'd known in London and Paris in the swinging sixties when he first found the fashion world at his feet.

I was glad, for the sake of a valued old friendship, that he didn't say the same to me and told me only that I was looking well and, true to form, he said: "By God, you need a haircut!" I had to laugh. You can't beat a London Cockney kid – even an old mate like Vidal – when it comes to keeping the cash registers jingling. He'd just rushed in from a work-out at a nearby gymnasium after a hectic weekend party at Playboy King Hugh Hefner's Bunny Lodge home.

"Have some herb tea," said Vidal, apologising for keeping me waiting – he'd got caught up in a Presidential motorcade – as he scooped out honey into two cups in the massive glass and chrome executive suite in Beverley Hills, from where he now runs his multi-million, international hairdressing empire. "Much better for you than ordinary tea with milk and sugar," he said, handing me the pale, yellow, sweet and scented brew. Then he sat back to talk about youth, health and longevity in the one city in the world in which, shallow though it may seem, life still revolves around sex and beauty and being seen to look good.

Hollywood, despite the depression of the last two decades, is still the home of most major movie-making and most of the famous television series which keep millions of people glued to the goggle box each night. The competition continues to be as enormous as it ever was. It is still the bitchiest, cruelest, most insecure place in the world. It's no wonder then that most of the men and women who live there worry more about their looks and spend more per capita on improving them, or hanging on to them, than in any other comparable international city. Their insecurity is scarcely surprising. Try to rattle off the names of ten stars of fifteen years ago who are still at the peak of the big time. It's hard.

It's a world, however, that suits Vidal right down to the toes of his expensive Gucci shoes. He has always been a glamour boy ever since he first emerged as a name in the early sixties in the swinging London of that era, and started socking his Geometric haircuts to the trendy set to become the hairdressing success story of all time. A rags-to-riches style story of the Cockney kid who left school at fourteen and had to get elocution lessons to get his first job in hairdressing. Until, says Vidal wryly today, "David Bailey came along two decades later and made being a Cockney okay."

His preoccupation today with health and longevity, vitality and the inner self is not just a new "in" fad that came along with his white Rolls Royce, his millionaire home with its star-sized pool in Beverley Hills which he shares with his beautiful actress wife, Beverly, and four small children.

"I was first turned on to this health thing in London twenty-five years ago," he says. Working a seventy hour week building up his business, often cutting hair from eight-thirty in the morning through to eight or ten at night, he found he was often feeling exhausted by late afternoon.

"Funnily enough," he says, "I think it was a client who suggested I try wheat germ."

In those days very little had been heard about wheat germ. But Vidal, game for anything, whipped up his first energy breakfast of wheat germ, yoghurt, raw eggs and honey. "We didn't even have blenders then, although it seems hard to believe, and it was all a bit of a giggle." But giggle or not, the health breakfast did really start to give him something he didn't have before – a new energy, a sort of "charge". Even fifteen years ago, anyone on a vegetarian diet or health foods was regarded, even in London, as a bit of a freak. Today, anyone looking at Vidal has to admit maybe the guy did have something after all. Certainly he has stuck with and expanded his philosophies on the way to feed and treat his body.

"There has to be something in it," he says. "I look at some of my friends in London who haven't lived, don't do anything. It's not that they're lazy, it's just that they haven't trained themselves to anything. They just get their feet up and they look ten or fifteen years older. Some of them look like my father." Perhaps they should take a leaf out of the Sassoon life style before it's too late, if they have the energy to start! At least four times a week – every day if possible – Vidal starts his day at five in the morning with a two and a half mile run. Then it's home for a quick shower followed by a dozen stretching exercises for fifteen minutes. A number of Vidal's friends, including actor, George Hamilton, often join him on the early morning run round the University of Southern California track. Sometimes a group of people will join in doing the exercises. Then comes the now, highly refined, health breakfast. Here is one of Vidal's recipes if you would like to try. He has adapted it to three hundred and sixty-five variations, one for every day of the year.

Protein Drink (Serves 2)

2 tablespoons powdered protein (from health food store or pharmacy)
1 tablespoon granula lecithin (from health food store or pharmacy)
1 large banana
1 raw egg
2 cups low-fat or skim milk
Toss everything into the blender and let it whip up for 30 seconds.

"After all that," says Vidal, "I go to work really on top of the world. You are charged up because the body machine needs the right fuel to energise itself. I think we all recognise this now. I try to make an analogy – you wouldn't fly in an aeroplane with second rate fuel. Of course not, you'd risk your life yet you risk your life every day by eating junk food."

When he arrived in California, Vidal found that many of the interesting, high energy people he met and worked with, all had the same approach to their food and health care. Take Carol Channing – one of the many stars who relied upon Vidal to do her hair and wigs. When Carol travels overseas she takes an enormous wardrobe and dozens of wigs. Vidal once spent four days with her in a New York hotel just cutting them. And guess what she packs, too. All her food, pre-packaged and prepared for her tour. She would never trust hotel or restaurant meals, so much importance does she place on what goes into the body machine in order to keep it in peak condition.

In the past the great stars always relied on the magic of the Hollywood make-up artists to see them through their middle years. As Vidal says, a good make-up job can make you look seventeen if you are forty if that's how the studio wants you to look for a part. So the stars didn't worry over much about their looks. They'd go out boozing the night before a big scene, get up looking like death in the morning and just stagger into the studio and the make-up artist's chair. Today views and attitudes to looks and health have radically changed. People are no longer looking to make-up to repair the ravages. Instead, they look within themselves for the way to look and feel younger all the time. Says Vidal, "They really want the knowledge – but at the moment they are having to fly around the world or cross the borders to Mexico or Chile to get it. It should be right here in this city. One day it will be."

The stars, of course, have always been patients at the famous cell therapy clinics. Niehans, at one point, would treat only the rich and famous, stars, royalty, Popes and Presidents. Many scores of famous names head, too, each year for Aslan's Fountain of Youth.

But what else, I wanted to know, was necessary to keep that enviable fantastic golden Californian look! Vidal is firm in his belief: "The only way to grow old gracefully is to be involved emotionally with your own body." And that doesn't mean you have to be a narcissist.

I recalled the woman overseas telegram operator who, on hearing me dictating a message explaining the book to Dr Stein in Germany, couldn't restrain herself. "I don't know about all that, dear," she said in a broad Australian accent, "I'm fat and nearly forty with six children and my family like me just the way I am."

Until now people didn't really have much choice, did they?

At the moment health food shops are mushrooming everywhere in California. People are all into buying healthier food and educating their children into better eating habits. I predict this will be universal within two to three years. Where Los Angeles goes first so the world trendies follow tomorrow.

One difference between the Hollywood Beautiful People and the rest of us is their dedication to exercise, meditation and yoga. A subscription to a health club is a must for every with-it girl. A man calls into his gym or uses private work-out facilities at home with the same matter-of-fact attitude the rest of us apply to a visit to our doctor, dentist or the supermarket. There are at least two places in the Beverley Hills area where you can go and take a full hour and a half of yoga. There are other gyms where you can lose weight, others, which I would adore, where you can spend ninety minutes working out with all the equipment dancers use so you can really get that Cyd Charisse or Shirley MacLaine flexibility in your body. I don't know where you could get it locally but I'm sure if a group of interested men or women approached a local theatre or night school something in the way of classes could be arranged. Vidal is a dedicated advocate of the use of both yoga and exercise. His wife Beverly is a yoga expert and the whole family, Catya, 19, Elan, nine, David, six and a half and baby of the family Eden, six, all swim and ride bicycles together. On longevity, Vidal believes the normal age will be one hundred – a healthy one hundred.

"There'll be a break-through sooner or later in finding the perfect youth cure but in the meantime, once people learn not to abuse their bodies, I see no reason why we shouldn't reach the one hundred mark."

One of Vidal's favourite treatments for himself is *fasting*. Every two weeks he fasts for thirty-six hours.

"I feel marvellous after it. It's a terrific feeling not having any food in your stomach. All tight and very light. I drink masses of bottled water, spring water while I'm fasting."

Transcendental meditation, too, is one of Vidal's recommendations for the really fit man or woman. Vidal met the Maharishi about fifteen years ago in a little hotel in Victoria, London, long before the Beatles and Mia Farrow became interested.

"He's an incredible man, an extraordinary man. He's so persuasive you really feel you have to meditate; to use the system because he has such an aura. I've been doing it for years and got back into it lately. When I am on the road putting on shows – (Vidal puts on international hair fashion extravaganzas) – as the pressure mounts I always meditate." The recommended twenty minutes night and morning, he says, is ideal, but he may do it for an hour or two.

What else do the Hollywood Beautiful People get up to on the quiet, to help them hang on to their good looks?

Vidal looked at me for a moment as if debating whether to spill the beans: "Well, there is bloodwashing in Mexico. Both George

Hamilton and I have been down there to give it a try."
  I couldn't wait to get on the youth trail to Tijuana . . .

CHAPTER FOURTEEN

The Quest for Youth In Mexico, Chile, And New Caledonia

"Ageing is an illness – not a fact of life"

Dr Jose Froimovich,
President Chilean Society of Gerontology

As the black Chevrolet with the dark tinted windows slid to a halt beside me in the main street of Tijuana, I heaved a sigh of relief. The man who climbed out or, rather, unwound himself from behind the driving wheel, was so tall, tanned and commanding he could only have been the youth doctor whom I had travelled three hundred miles that morning to see. Leaving before breakfast, I had driven from the seething high rise fantasy world of Hollywood to this seedy fly-blown Mexican border town.

Tijuana, just a rumbling cart track and half-finished concrete roadway from the high speed modern artery of the South California freeway to San Diego, is one of the world's havens for doctors who practice on the fringe of conventional medicine. Only a few miles across the border they are able to run their clinics in comparative peace despite officials of the high powered American Food and Drug Administration, who spend their days buzzing, like so many angry flies, harassing patients on the border in a stable door attempt to discourage trade.

Judging by the thousands of patients who flock to the Mexican clinics annually – many suffering from incurable diseases; Parkinsons disease, cancer, muscular dystrophy and other circulatory and heart diseases, officialdom is failing dismally.

My goal on this occasion, a hot summers day, was not to see the cancer clinics but to find out all there was to know about the youth doctor about whom so many of the famous are talking. And to discover what his revolutionary bloodwashing and youth treatments involve.

Count Anthony Roman Schenk, M.D. Ph.D., Knight Commander of the Order of St. John – according to his expensive looking gilded business card – has been practicing medicine for thirty-five years. He has been in Mexico for over twenty of them.

Trying to track him down was a feat in itself. Nobody, from the stars who number among his clients to the secretary who had driven her sick father there the previous weekend, seemed to know the precise address. The phone number rarely answered or, when it did, a tinny Mexican voice, which sounded as if it came from the moon, repeated with boring obstinacy that Dr Schenk was not available.

All of those, who seemed as anxious as I was that we should meet, were quite clear about the point in the middle of Tijuana where I should find the clinic. Which is how I came to be waiting for half an hour, according to instructions, beside a red plastic statue of a tennis player in Tijuana's sleezy main street.

Was I on a wild goose chase after all, I was asking myself for the twentieth time as I squinted in both directions for the dark coloured Chevrolet in which Dr Schenk had assured me he would come and find me.

Introductions over, we drove off in a cloud of dust up a winding track to the Villa Caliente – a large pink stucco house overlooking the township. Dr Schenk unlocked the high gate and led me past a swimming pool over a marble terrace. Crisp, dried leaves rustled across it in the slight breeze which didn't reach the burning dust streets of the town below.

"The marble lights up, underneath, at night to form a dance floor" the Doctor told me as he led the way in. He said he was sorry about the leaves – his houseboy was away.

With the hospitality of the Middle European, he poured cool, white wine, as he settled me comfortably in the velvet chairs in his drawing room. I was indeed honoured. Not many of Dr Schenk's visitors ever see his private home – a haven where an inner courtyard is flanked by his laboratory and rooms for visiting doctors. My eyes, as he began talking, were constantly drawn to a large painting on the dining room wall of the devil, well horned, a giant syringe and an ace of spades.

"Yes," said the Doctor reading my question, "I have studied under three African witchdoctors in my time."

He also says he has a Ph.D in Biochemistry, to have been an internist in Germany, to have done a Post Graduate course in Endocyinology in Austria and, finally, to have become involved in Gerontology as an assistant to the famous cell therapist, Paul Niehans, at his clinic in Switzerland.

"My main interest is in old age diseases – diseases which don't respond to any treatment," which is one of the main reasons why Dr Schenk receives so many calls from no hopers, terminal patients at the end of their tether looking for a miracle. And why his methods for the most part have had to remain on the wrong side of the Mexican border – wrong side as far as acceptance by the American F.D.A is concerned, with their stringent rules over proper testing of every drug and treatment that comes within ten feet of any patient.

Whether Dr Schenk has any successes I cannot tell you. I only know that whatever he does is sufficiently successful for scores of patients to take the rough road to his clinic, sometimes every ten days, and drive the three hundred miles from Los Angeles and further afield because they believe it has something for them.

Certainly, in checking as thoroughly as possible on the medical grapevine in the U.S. and Europe it would seem that Dr Schenk's claim is true, that he has never caused harm to any patient through his treatments, however revolutionary.

"I have not had a failure," said Dr Schenk. Certainly none of his patients has ever died as a direct result of his treatment.

Bloodwashing is the basis of all Dr Schenk's treatments, in his word the "perfectionment" of the system, a purifying process.

It doesn't, as the imagination prompts, involve transfusions of the blood. It is an injection treatment called Sulconar using vaccines, anti-toxins and other enzymes. It was developed by Professor Morrison in Buenos Aires in Argentina.

Explaining his treatment Dr Schenk says: "What is the good of trying to treat a system that is not first of all purified, cleared out of all toxins? Otherwise one is covering up the root cause of many of the problems." The bloodwashing treatment, he says, lowers cholesterol levels, reduces the blood pressure and removes residual bacteria infection in the arteries.

"If anybody has hereditary factors such as poor circulation or arteriosclerosis then no rejuvenation treatment can possibly help until he has put his cardiovascular system in order."

Schenk claims that in three or four treatments a patient's cardiovascular system can be improved by fifteen to twenty years. The whole of his philosophy seems to be a back to nature attempt to undo the damage of everyday living, and to restore the system to as near perfect a condition as possible.

Nevertheless, Dr Schenk is extremely secretive about his methods and his injections are imported from Argentina by various devious routes. Patients come to the clinic from all over the world, all over the U.S. and from Europe. The secretary I met in Los Angeles had been regularly taking her bed-ridden father who was suffering from Parkinsons Disease. "He swears by the doctor's treatment," she told me. "He believes the doctor holds out the only hope for him. He seems a little better each time we go there but we know it is going to be very slow."

Claims Dr Schenk: "Most chronic diseases which are untouchable with conventional methods can be cured, because by purifying the system you take the cause of the disease away."

However, he did stress this did not apply to cancerous diseases, sclerosis or blindness. Dr Schenk was loathe to talk about his rejuvenation programme, but according to Vidal Sasson, large numbers of Hollywood stars and American businessmen do trek to Tijuana regularly to have the purifying jabs which will put their cells back in order and a sparkle back in their life style.

As I left the Villa Caliente and waved goodbye I was conscious of a great loneliness in the tall figure standing behind the gate. The youth business has been for many, certainly among the older practitioners, a solitary road.

Anthony Schenk can be contacted through: Specialised Medical Services, P.O. Box 1995, 1315 San Ysidro, California, 92073, U.S.A.

Dr Schenk is not the only youth doctor in Mexico – far from it. There are numerous clinics claiming to have found the elixir of long life, health and beauty. It is also a haven in particular for cancer treatments. In the course of my travels and researches I became quite closely drawn in to their problems and intrigued by some of their success stories. I will tell you about them when I discuss cancer and its relation to the ageing problem.

But from Mexico I took a look at yet another of the clinics attracting the Hollywood stars – this time in Chile . . .

Doctor Jose Froimovich of Santiago, Chile is a man who claims to have developed a youth drug which can enable anyone to live to the age of one hundred and twenty. He is one of the many doctors who now believe that people should live normally to be between one hundred and one hundred and twenty years – as nature intended.

Froimovich, one of the most respected South American gerontological researchers, has been delving into the problems of ageing for over thirty-six years – to find a way of slowing down the ageing process. With the help of an enormous team of scientists in Chile – over ninety doctors, chemists and medical specialists – he came up with the drug he has claimed could provide a universal answer.

His formula is called FGF-60 – mainly because it consists of a combination of sixty vitamins, hormones, minerals and extracts of organs all of which are necessary to retard ageing. The treatment is given in capsule form, one type specially for women and one for men, each of which differ in hormone content. The male pills, for example, obviously contain no female hormones and vice versa.

Dr Froimovich maintains that his capsules are a synthesis of all the products the human body no longer secretes after a certain age. The treatment has been tested over the years on hundreds of volunteer elderly patients – and in one series of clinical tests in ninety-two physical categories all critical to ageing, every one of the "guinea pig" patients showed improvements in one or more areas. Some showed better results than others depending on their disabilities to start with.

For example, somebody hard of hearing may have shown a seventy per cent increase improvement while you could hardly show a positive result if you weren't deaf in the first place. However, the doctor believes that all people would benefit from his formula in some way.

Dr Froimovich says that it is possible for his treatment to slow the ageing process down sufficiently well to allow a man easily to reach his genetic age of one hundred and twenty years. FGF-60, he claims, can *reverse* the process of ageing. And, he says, it *can* help people to see and hear a little better, and give them more virility and strength enabling them to enjoy their sex life better.

It will also, he says, prevent many of the diseases of ageing such as circulatory and heart problems, strokes and heart attacks. And if he is to be believed, wrinkles can be seen to lessen, skin becomes smoother, hair stops falling out and energy increases tremendously. In many cases people who can no longer walk when they arrive at his clinic end up not only walking but running after treatment! I can't endorse that as I haven't seen the results. But I did receive first hand reports from one of three partners in a firm called Selfco Inc. in Wilshire Boulevard, Beverley Hills, California, who intend to market FGF-60 in the United States and internationally before too long, and hope it will become available over the chemist's counter.

Dafna Edwards is blonde, young and extremely glamorous and works in television. Yes, she said, she has also had FGF-60 so there was no point in asking her age. Dafna was living in a pretty little house in Los Angeles with a huge white dog and three girlfriends. Her interest in Dr Froimovich began when her late husband suffering from leukaemia went there, as a last resort, to seek treatment.

He couldn't be treated. As Dafna says, he was "too far gone," but after his death his young widow became fascinated by the work of the clinic.

"I have seen people who have gone down there," she says, "and couldn't even walk. Afterwards they've thrown their canes away. Others have gone there with arthritis and they are dancing today. I have seen people come back who thought they were dying beforehand. It is just incredible . . ."

She describes a film which was made comparatively recently documenting the progress of some of Dr Froimovich's patients in the Santiago clinic. It shows them entering the clinic on crutches and wheelchairs. Some are suffering from Parkinson's Disease, others from arthritis or just old age deterioration and dehydration, and some of them can't even walk at all. After treatment you see the same patients miraculously walking, exercising and even running around. Some run four hundred to eight hundred metres and even play basketball. Dr Froimovich believes man should be allowed to live healthily with full mental and physical capacity for his full life span – as he was originally programmed to do. The idea of the Froimovich formula is to bring man up to his genetic age of 120. Animals, he says, live to their full genetic age, man does not, due to all the chemicals with which he fills his body. Froimovich is described by an associate as a human computer, a genius. Throughout the last three decades he has channelled all the work done by his team of scientists into one direction – the perfection of his formula.

First of all, way back in 1939, he induced artifical old age in animals, laboratory mice, rats and rabbits, through surgical procedures as well as adding foods like egg yoke, cholesterol, plain eggs and dried bovine marrow to their food, which at that time was thought to be consistent with producing arteriosclerosis.

After obtaining symptoms typical of ageing, Froimovich tried to retrogress them by using procedures already tried by youth doctors like Brown-Sequard, Voronoff and Bogomoletz before him, by transplanting testicles, ovaries and injecting connective tissues. His purpose was to establish the concept that old age and its symptoms could be artifically produced and could also be reversed back to the original healthy state. This he undeniably did. For the next ten years at the Laboratory of Experimental Medicine in Chile, he had a team of ten scientists performing over fifty thousand biochemical tests to determine the changes that take place in the blood, urine, tissues and organs during the development of the human organism right through maturity to old age.

Examinations started from the age of six to ten years right through to 110 years old. On each of the guinea pig subjects, 74 tests were carried out to measure and compare the substance of the human body such as proteins, iron, vitamins, hormones, sodium and nitrogen. While some substances diminished others increased depending upon the age of the subject. The resulting conclusions formed the basis of the doctor's present day formula.

In the fourth period of his work Froimovich turned to research into the complex functions of the liver and lipotrism. After all these years of painstaking research Froimovich reached the stage of being able to apply his treatment to human beings in their fight against ageing. Over 15,000 tests were performed on 150 men and women and the results were presented to the Gerontological Society of Chile.

Finally 162 old people were selected as patients for his FGF-60 treatment. The 131 men had an average age of seventy-four and 31 women had an average age of 75.3. All of them had no serious illnesses and were intelligent enough to answer questions. After examination by 62 professionals in different medical fields, the patients were subjected to 92 clinical, instrumental and laboratory tests. Every one of them showed improvement in one or more areas, after treatment.

The results of Dr Froimovich's work have been carefully documented over the years in scores of medical papers as well as being presented by him at numerous medical congresses and, as a respected medical researcher, his articles have appeared in some of the world's most prestigious medical journals. In 1968 he won the John R. Reitemeyer Award presented by the International Press Soceity in Buenos Aires, Argentina for outstanding medical journalism. In Washington D.C. at the Eighth International Congress of Gerontology, Dr Froimovich presented a complete report of his three year tests on the 162 patients to whom he gave the FGF-60 treatments. What does the treatment involve?

Patients first of all have blood and physical tests to determine any ailments. Next they begin a two week course of hormone pills and plenty of exercise. Exercise is important in order to activate the body machinery and improve circulation.

Says Dafna Edwards: "The formula will work if you are in bed but it will not work as well as if you exercise." Miss Edwards spoke of long walks over the Chilean hills with the elusive actress Greta Garbo while she was undergoing treatment there. "A wonderful, delightful woman."

Diet, too, plays an important part in the treatment. For example, Dr Froimovich is totally against patients eating eggs, and he refuses to let anybody eat meat because of its high cholesterol content. This is only during the treatment period, but afterwards the doctor advises a nutritious vegetarian diet.

At present the doctor has agreed to submit his findings to the U.S. Senate Special Committee on Ageing, an approval which could greatly help in easing FGF-60 through the Food and Drug Administration who will, of course, have to approve the treatment before it can be offered for sale in the U.S.

Meanwhile, according to gerontologists like Dr Froimovich a fifty year increase in our life expectancy is quite possible by the year 1990 and by the middle of the 21st Century he agrees it might be quite normal to live to be two hundred.

So there you are – more evidence on my road to Shangri-La. A French doctor who practices in Noumea, New Caledonia, off the north-east coast of Australia, has a different use for cell therapy. He claims that by injecting fresh cells directly into facial wrinkles he can make the wrinkles completely vanish for up to a year.

What concerned me was what happens at the end of the year – would you wake up one morning to find the wrinkles had suddenly, horrifically, popped back into place?

According to the doctor, who launched his discovery amongst society women in Paris, there is no need for such fears. The wrinkles would gently ease their way back in the same way that they appeared in the first place. The treatment is especially devised for wrinkles under and around the eyes.

Unfortunately, once again I cannot name the doctor, due to French medical ethics which forbid qualified, practicing doctors to indulge in publicity. However, he talked to me at some length about his treatments and I met women who had tried it.

The doctor says the best results are obtained on people aged between thirty and fifty-five. Even an old face, however, can be made to look much younger as a result of the injections. The treatment is based on the theory of cell therapy in which the fresh cells, in this case deep frozen and flown from France, obtained from unborn lambs assist in regenerating the cells of the facial skin which start flagging due to age.

One of the biggest problems of ageing is the loss of elasticity in the skin which causes sagging and bagging and ultimately wrinkles. The doctor's magic wrinkle treatment consists of a series of injections using a special, extremely fine needle, every millimetre along the length of the wrinkle. All the injections are given at the same time. A spray on local anaesthetic in the area of the operation removes any pain or discomfort during the injections.

Afterwards, patients are told to remain in their room for one day and for six days to be as quiet as possible to rest the facial muscles. The doctor says it is extremely effective, causes a new firming up and tightening of the skin as well as a new bloom to the complexion.

Many patients have had the wrinkle treatment in conjunction with general cell therapy.

CHAPTER FIFTEEN

Bio-Stimulated Egg Therapy

"We must aim to prevent disease rather than merely relieve symptoms."

Dr Ivan M. Popov, Nassau

Bio-stimulated egg therapy is the high-faluting name applied to the curious treatment given to patients at the Renaissance Revitalization Center in Nassau in the Bahamas.

Fertilised chicken eggs are swallowed by patients anxious to achieve rejuvenation. According to the clinic, which is run by the famed rejuvenator Dr Ivan M. Popov, the eggs are used to supply embryonic foetal tissue to ageing tissues of the body. On the very doorstep of the youth-conscious United States, Popov's clinic is, of course, a mecca for ageing Americans.

According to Popov, the philosophy of Renaissance is to treat the total individual with a series of therapies that aim for good health and prevention of disease, rather than concentrating merely on relieving existing symptoms.

As in similar centres, the usual ten-day stay begins with individual examination of the patient, during which a programme of biological therapies is recommended as a top-to-toe stimulus to the system.

One of the main treatments at the centre is the Thalasso (Greek word meaning "sea") therapy, a treatment using the benefits of unpolluted sea water. Many centres around the world are already using this method to improve health and vitality, particularly in Romania where for centuries the spa waters have been found to be beneficial. The benefits of sea water therapy have been known in Europe since 1910 when the first experiments were conducted by a

Dr Quinton.

As Dr Popov's clinic explains it: "Since the proportion of trace elements in the sea is comparable to the same proportion of chemicals in human blood plasma, we know that any application of such elements is in consonance with body functioning."

The clinic gives thermal sea water pressure massages and showers to help improve the circulation, muscle tone and to gain absorption of microscopic biological elements into the system. They say that these treatments, combined with the inhaling of aerosolised sea water mist, and oxygen and aroma therapy, can help to detoxify the respiratory tract and provide stimulation to the body tissues.

Personally, I take all this with more than a pinch of sea salt. I reckon you can do as much good by doing as I do – adding a generous two ounces of sea salt from the grocers or chemists to your nightly bath. It's great for toning your body and marvellous for keeping winter scaly feet smooth!

Another treatment practised by Popov's medical team is sleep therapy which they say is based on over 25 years experience with sleep institutes throughout the Soviet Union. The idea is to reach a complete state of relaxation by touching on the neurological system associated with sleep. This can prove extremely beneficial to chronic insomniacs, many of whom find they can abandon sleeping pills and tranquillisers after treatment.

Clients at Renaissance have ranged from the age of 25 to their 90's and they usually stay at a nearby hotel on Cable Beach while undergoing treatment at the centre.

For further information you can write or telephone: Renaissance Revitalization Centre, Cable Beach, P.O. Box N4854, Nassau, Bahamas. (809) 32-78441-2.

CHAPTER SIXTEEN

The Rush For Vitamin B-15

"There is no room in science for belief. We deal in facts."
Dr Ernst T. Krebs, San Francisco,
Discoverer of the Youth Treatment B-15.

They have been giving Vitamin B-15 to racehorses and greyhounds for years to make them run faster. But when they offered it to a group of human guinea pigs in Sydney, Australia, as the latest youth cure, there was a several hundred-strong stampede down the plushy corridors of a leading city hotel, as eager men and women rushed to try it.

Today, only five years later, B-15 is already regarded by millions of people as their own breakfast-time mini-miracle in the fight against age. Each morning, along with their toast, cereals or orange juice they quickly swallow one or more of the tiny pills which look like aspirin, taste like chalk, contain minute quantities of cyanide and which are fast becoming the best-selling youth pill on the international market, under the innocent guise of a dietary health food.

True to its name – it is known technically as Pangamic Acid, from the word "pan" meaning "everywhere" and "gami", the word for "seed" – the origins of B-15 are somewhere in the kernel of the apricot stone. Thousands of those who take it claim that it makes them feel fitter and healthier and – most vital of all – makes them look ten to fifteen years younger due, they say, to its beneficial side-effects.

Yet, ironically, the men who market it find themselves in an impossible *Catch 22* situation – they want to cash in on the sales boom, but dare not publicise its rejuvenating properties for fear of a massive clamp down by already sceptical health authorities.

Its cause has not been helped by the way in which it has been confusingly linked with its sister treatment, B-17, the notorious cancer cure known as Laetrile, which also has its source in the apricot stone. Doubts over the safety of B-17, because of its cyanide content, have caused a continuing uproar across America, as a result of which Laetrile has been banned or is subject to legal restriction in many parts of the United States.

Similarly, conventional doctors and scientists in the U.S. and Britain, too, make no secret of the fact that they would like to see Vitamin B-15 banned because, although they agree it is harmless, they say it is also totally useless.

But in spite of this the Pangamate boom has continued to win increasing numbers of converts to its magical claims. To health faddist Americans B-15 has already become a trendy national obsession. Perhaps it is not too surprising that a nation already souped-up with daily vitamins should rush to clasp this latest panacea to their already pill-packed bosoms. Experts estimate that around 40 million Americans are on the vitamin bandwaggon and may well take well over 20 tablets a day, some may even take many more. Since B-15 became available over the counter in the United States – less than two years ago – manufacturers claim that several million American customers are using it regularly, clearing health stores from coast to coast of supplies of Pangamik 15 and other trade names, under which B-15 is sold.

Muhammad Ali, Burt Reynolds, Clint Walker and Senator Barry Goldwater, as well as the U.S. Show Jumping team, are among the many thousands who the manufacturers claim have already tried it. Ali is said to have started taking B-15 just before meeting Jimmy Young in his 1976 defence of the World Championship and continued with it during his fights with Richard Dunn and Ken Norton. He is said to be still on it today.

Yet, although B-15 was first discovered and developed in the United States over a quarter of a century ago by the brilliant and controversial San Francisco biochemist, Dr Ernst T. Krebs, Junior, it was rigidly banned from America until only recently. Krebs, himself, has fought a long and bitter battle with the American Food and Drug Administration to get them to accept that B-15 is a vitamin and not a drug in order to give thousands of Americans the opportunity of openly using it, instead of smuggling it in from the chemists of Europe as they have had to in the past. Now, perversely, the F.D.A. are saying that B-15 is not even a vitamin, but a food additive and they refuse point-blank to accept that it has any value at all.

In the meantime, people in Russia, Japan, Yugoslavia, Spain and Germany have long been reaping the benefits of B-15 for themselves.

In simple terms, B-15 is claimed by many scientists to have a definite effect in slowing down the ageing process. It helps increase the intake of oxygen into the blood and body tissues, thereby increasing the life-span of the cells and setting off a chain reaction of regenerative effects. The easiest way to understand it, say experts, is to think of it as instant oxygen which speeds detoxification of wastes and increases supplies of oxygen to every part of the body.

Russian scientists were among the first to decide that B-15 had indeed a wide and varied health potential. They researched and developed their own formula for B-15 which they export to many countries, as well as being manufactured under licence. After rigorously testing and recording the results of the effect of B-15 on people of all ages, particularly the aged, Russian scientists gave the go-ahead to the Soviet drug industry in 1968 to mass produce B-15 for general use. And in the 205-page symposium of their findings, the U.S.S.R. Academy of Sciences stated emphatically that B-15 is effective in retarding the signs of old age. They say that by far the most important effect is the oxygen absorption by the cells so increasing the cells' life-span and improving the functions of all the body organs – hence that feeling of vitality and well-being

For some considerable time the Russians have been giving the treatment to their own sportsmen, astronauts, athletes and gymnasts to help improve fitness and stamina. Also, thousands of ordinary Russians have been taking it for a number of years to increase health and longevity. In fact, it has become almost as common to see a bottle of Calcium Pangamate (B-15) on Russian meal tables, as it is for us to see pepper and salt. Indeed, one

Moscow doctor says he believes the time is not far distant when it will be an accepted part of every meal-time for all people over forty.

But despite all this it was not until the mid-1970's that the popular B-15 boom began, when a leading Australian cookery writer, Margaret Fulton, announced that at 51 she suddenly looked and felt a good decade younger. Her new recipe for success, she said, was a vitamin called B-15 which she had been receiving during a ten-injection course at a city slimming clinic. That did it! Switchboards were jammed, people wrote, telephoned and even arrived by the coach-load to avail themselves of what was reputed to be the latest in youth-giving treatments.

The treatment being given in Sydney was based on the Russian formula, which was being made in Australia under licence. Later, I interviewed a large number of patients, all of whom had taken the treatment in combined pill and injection form. They all used almost identical phrases in describing their feelings to me. They felt full of a new "joie de vivre", they had more energy, new exuberance and vitality and, best of all, everybody was telling them they looked a good ten to fifteen years younger. Margaret Fulton was even asked by one less-than-tactful friend if she had had a face-lift. She hadn't. But what more could anyone ask?

Let's take a look first at the views and reports of some of the ordinary men and women, the guinea-pigs, who were the first one hundred Australian patients to try B-15 for themselves.

Maggie Deas, a 35-year-old red-haired Australian model told me: "Frankly, I'm on it for the youth bit." As each day went past Maggie rang up with increasingly enthusiastic reports on her progress. At the start of the course she was pretty run-down, having been managing a restaurant for her husband and, with two children, was badly in need of a health boost. In the first week Maggie reported more energy and she told me, "I am glowing! I have never felt better in my life. My skin looks tauter, my hair – always in bad condition – has never looked better. Everybody I have met has asked me what I have been doing, and if they can do it, too. I feel on top of the world."

Another enthusiast was actress and singer Toni Lamond, in her early forties and sister of Australian international singing star, Helen Reddy. Toni investigated the background of the treatment carefully before embarking. However, after the course she was bubbling with its success. "I have suddenly become vain!" she laughed. "I am looking in mirrors for the first time in years and I know I am looking younger. The other day a T.V. viewer wrote in to ask if I had had a face–lift, and a 23-year-old young man apparently found me attractive the other night. Very good for the ego when you have a son in his twenties." Toni reported a new elasticity in her skin and added, "Today, with the accent on youth fads, none of us dare to grow old. And if B-15 can help – I say great!"

Another beautician I interviewed said she had received seven injections to date, spread out twice weekly, and was taking additional B-15 tablets morning and evening. "At the end of the first week I began to feel extra energy and a sense of well-being and good health. When I sit down in the evenings after a hard day I am not tired. There's no tension, nothing I wouldn't tackle. I also find my palate has changed. I used to love potatoes – now I don't like them." She, too, found friends and clients commenting on her looks. People were asking her what she had done to herself. "I am certainly looking more youthful, but it could be due to feeling so well. Even my hair is bouncy again."

This particular beautician believes from her experience that ageing goes in steps or plateaus gradually downwards from puberty. She theorises that the vitamin treatment can hold you where you are for a longer period before your body continues the ageing process. She reported on another client of hers who had taken B-15. "She had a sallowish, yellow skin for years – now it is clear again," she says.

Margaret Fulton, who was among the very first to try the cure, says she didn't originally try it as a rejuvenation treatment, but as a sort of "topping-off" of her slimming treatment. She didn't even tell her husband she intended to try it – she was so busily involved in her career at the time. Then, she said, people began to comment and ask her what she had been doing to herself. "Everywhere they were saying how marvellous I looked, and the man at my delicatessen even jokingly asked if I had been on a youth pill." My husband made a point of saying how pretty I looked when I had been out gardening, and my daughter said my skin looked even better these days without make-up. I realised then that I had been letting myself go. I had been looking at myself through rose coloured glasses for years. Even my husband admitted he thought I was trying to turn myself into an old woman before my time. Men are making passes at me for the first time in years."

One of the most exciting moments was when actor, Danny Kaye, took special notice of her at a luncheon for cookery writers. "But," said Margaret frankly, "Men making passes at me, and my husband telling me I look pretty are minor things compared to the wonderful way I feel. There's a sort of joyousness in doing things again. I've got this wonderful feeling of well-being."

One of the most satisfying and useful side-effects of vitamin B-15 is as a hangover cure. It's found to be one of the best remedies yet. In fact, one doctor told me you can drink two bottles of wine, take a shot of B-15 and in two hours you will be back to normal – sober as a judge.

The rush to Pangamic Acid in Australia caused alarm among the cagey and careful Australian health authorities, who closely follow the guidelines of their American cousins in the F.D.A. in clamping down quickly on anything about which they don't know enough. B-15 came into this category and curiously and silently within a few weeks, after a few tentative enquiries by the men from the Ministry, chemists manufacturing the injections and pills suddenly found their sources of raw material – all imported – had dried up. Supplies on the docks were just not being unloaded. But, meanwhile, the word was spreading around the world and so was B-15!

Since its arrival over the counter in the U.S.A. it was only a matter of time before it slipped through Britain's back door, too. It is now selling in health food stores and by mail order under a silent cloud of disapproval from health authorities. However, say the U.K. manufacturers who sell it guardedly under the label of a natural diet food, as long as they take care not to make any claims for it at all, they feel the authorities will continue to turn a blind eye.

But, say the manufacturers, "B–15 is only just beginning to be known in Britain. It is all still pretty low key – people who want it can get it from health food stores, but they still have to search for it or send for it by mail order."

Most of the supplies are being manufactured in Britain with added apricot kernel powder (B–17) in the formula. Other varieties being sold are imported from Puerto Rico and Germany. Russian biochemists report their most fantastic results with B–15 have been when it was combined with Ginseng.

One of the best-selling over-the-counter combinations in Britain is B–15 Plus – a formula which contains Siberian Ginseng, B–15, Vitamin B–6 and Vitamin B–13, the trace element Zinc. One of the first people to try it was the rejuvenation and health expert, the famous author Barbara Cartland, herself a glamorous and youthful septegenarian.

The man they call "The Father of Laetrile," the scientist who discovered it, Krebs, is the biochemist at the very heart of America's bitter cancer cure war – over B–17 – the Laetrile cancer treatment. It was as long ago as 1952 that Krebs found B–15 almost as an accidental by-product while he was researching into the chemical properties of the apricot kernel to determine the active principle in his cancer cure. Dr Krebs never fails to emphasise that although both substances spring from the same mysterious life-giving apricot seed, there the similarity ends.

In the midst of the tangled web of controversy surrounding the youth pill (B–15) and the even more politically explosive Laetrile (B–17), it is interesting to look at the man himself and the deep scientific dedication of the mind behind these two discoveries. Dr Krebs is a big, blond hulk of a man – quiet, shy, gentlemanly and aloof. A strict German Lutheran by religion, like his father before him – also an eminent scientist – he began his adult career with the intention of following in his father's footsteps into medicine. He even enrolled in medical school, but as time went by he became convinced that his future lay, not in the everyday care of the health of his patients, but in the deep and more complex world of medical chemistry.

So Krebs became, not a doctor of medicine, but after three years of anatomy and medicine at the Hahnemann Medical College in Philadelphia, he became a Doctor of Biochemistry. His undergraduate career was intriguing and brilliant. He spent much of it at the Universtiy of Illinois from 1938 to 1941, specialising in Bacteriology and receiving his Bachelor's Degree in 1942. He later went on to do graduate work at the University of California from 1943 to 1945. Later, he researched in Pharmacology at the University of Mississippi and he has received numerous international doctorates and honours for his work.

Today Krebs is acknowledged as one of the world's most formidable biochemists as well as a remarkable theologian and a warm and deeply concerned human being, although he prefers to give the impression of the fierce and remote scientist who suffers no fools.

His beautiful, large, old, family mansion in the historic Mission district of San Francisco – one of the few old houses in the area remaining in its original form – is a Mecca for doctors and academics who come to learn at his table from all over the world. An audience with Dr Krebs is, indeed, to be called to the court of one of the most amazing brains of our times. One of the greatest values in meeting him is to hear some of his vast knowledge in relation to health and nutrition, particularly today. He speaks fast and vehemently in staccato American tones of his theories and beliefs.

I arrived at the old panelled house with its giant entrance hall housing the family's church organ, to be asked peremptorily where my luggage was "Why haven't you come to stay?"

I was ushered into the book-lined drawing room and told I would have twenty minutes with the Master. More discussions would be held over lunch – egg sandwiches and ice-cream – in the magnificent dining hall with its church stained-glass windows and dark panelling.

Krebs' own description of B-15 is to think of it as instant oxygen. It detoxifies the liver as a transmethylating agent and helps to increase the oxygen intake of all the tissues, causing a regenerative reaction. As a result, although it is not proven, Krebs believes that B-15 is indirectly an anti-cancer agent.

As I have pointed out, B-15 is particularly well accepted by the

Russians, especially for Russian athletes, who are reported to have been administered with heavy doses of B-15 during recent Olympic Games. The reasons for this are fairly evident: facts show that the vitamin, although a natural food, can greatly increase physical stamina.

One Russian experiment, using rats placed in barrels of water, showed that the animals which had been treated with Pangamic Acid (B-15) were able to swim long after the rest had drowned from exhaustion.

Extensive clinical tests carried out by the Russians on teams of aged patients showed also that B-15 is effective in the treatment of many diseases such as heart conditions, circulatory problems, high blood cholesterol, some skin disorders, diabetes, hardening of the arteries, bronchial and respiratory problems and in accelerating the healing of wounds as well as soothing nerves and lessening tension. Their reports concluded that B-15 was most beneficial in retarding the ageing process.

It is fascinating to note that in Hunza in the Himalayas where people frequently live to over 100, and often 120, their diet contains large quantities of fresh and dried apricots, and it is not uncommon to eat 30-50 apricot seeds as an after-dinner snack. Also, cancer is unknown in Hunza.

One of Doctor Krebs' greatest problems today is to try to clarify the confusion between his two inventions: B-15, which is slowly winning ground as a youth and rejuvenation treatment and which is in no way being claimed as a cancer cure; and his highly controversial Amygdalin (Vitamin B-17, or Laetrile), which is still the subject of a major battle to legalise it in the United States.

At the time of going to print B-17 was legalised under State legislation in Alaska, Indiana, Florida, Arizona, Nevada, Texas, Washington, Oklahoma, Delaware, Lousiana, New Hampshire, Oregon, Illinois, New Jersey, Kansas, Idaho, Maryland, North Dakota and Montana.

One of his closest aides says: "The trouble is that the Government agencies have tried to tar B-15, which is not used for cancer, but which is used all over the world to retard the process of ageing, with the same brush as B-17, this trying to get both treatments outlawed."

Krebs is the portly hub-pin at the centre of this wheel of controversy, the tracks of which cut deep and dirty over the last decade as it careered across the muddy playing fields of U.S. politics. With a quiet dignity, Krebs has kept himself withdrawn from most of his explosive attackers when, less than 5 years ago, with Laetrile (B-17) under total ban, it was branded as "godamn quackery" by many of his fiercest critics.

At present B-17 is known to be used by over 50,000 American cancer victims, as well as by many patients in Europe, the Philippines, Britain and Australia. Krebs' dearest wish is to see Laetrile finally legalised.

In a major breakthrough in the last two years, Laetrile has been legalised at Federal level for "all those who have cancer or believe they have cancer" provided patient and physician sign a standard affidavit for its acquisition. And if Krebs and his followers win a "Laetrile case" currently before the United States Supreme Court, Laetrile will become legal in all 50 states without restriction to its users.

There are numerous claims that, in some way, regular doses of B-17 have prevented cancer from increasing and, in fact, retards the symptoms even in some cases causing them to disappear. I met one woman patient in her 60's. She was slim, grey-haired and attractive. She had terminal cancer 30 years ago in Dr Krebs' father's day. She told me she had been put on regular doses of Vitamin B-17 and the cancer had disappeared. In recent years she stopped taking it – and the cancer started up again. Today, on her regular dosages of several apricot kernels a day, she is a healthy and energetic secretary.

Another man I met was given 5 years to live by his doctor, having had every operation possible to save him. His case, he was told, was terminal . . . hopeless. Today, although his face is lined and creased with the suffering of the past, his eyes are bright and twinkling with hope and enjoyment of each new day. His cancer is being held at bay and he spends his time working to help legalise the drug and so benefit others.

Another terminal cancer victim on the brink of death, himself a doctor, reported how he previously refused to believe in Laetrile. Then, as a final resort, he gave himself a massive dose of B-17 almost as his last dice to try and cheat death. To his amazement he found the pain receding and his appetite returning. Within three months he was able to return to work.

Hundreds of doctors are studying the effects or taking the treatment themselves. There are moves to open factories to produce B-17 in Australia, and it is already being made in Germany and Britain. European distributors are also importing from Mexico.

The problem, as far as health authorities are concerned, is that Laetrile or Amygdalin is obtained from the crushed kernel of the apricot stone – which contains cyanide – and the biggest question that arises for the fearful, the ignorant and the layman is simply the obvious one. Is Laetrile poisonous?

What exactly are the dangers of that cyanide content? According to Krebs Junior and respected biochemists working with him, there is no question of doubt at all: Laetrile, they say, is a non-toxic compound and can safety be given to patients in large doses for long periods.

Krebs, who carried on his research into B-17 from his father, and a team of hospital doctors who worked on the theory in the late 20's and 30's, discovered that it was Amygdalin that was the active substance in curing cancer rather than the apricot kernel enzymes themselves. And he found that the active and vital part of the Amygdalin was the cyanide portion of the molecule.

Krebs was convinced that Laetrile was not poisonous. The molecule contained two units of glucose, one of benzaldehyde and one of cyanide, all tightly locked in together. But there is only one enzyme in the body which can unlock the dangerous cyanide and that is beta-glucosidase, and although that is to be found in most parts of the body it is only present on a danger or "unlocking" level at or around cancerous cells. Which, in lay terms, means that the cyanide in B-17 could only be released directly onto the cancer cells. To counterbalance the smaller amounts of the unlocking enzyme the body contains, in all areas except around cancer cells, a protective enzyme called rhodanese will cloak the "unlocking" enzyme and neutralise the cyanide, converting it into health giving and regenerative by-products.

To prove it was safe to use B-17 on humans, Krebs first injected it into his own body in 1950 – with no ill effects. He then tried it on his first cancer patients.

Dr Dean Burk, formerly Chief Chemist in the Department of Cell Chemistry at the National Cancer Institute in Washington, wrote in 1972 quite categorically on the safety of Laetrile. He has this to say:

"With 45 years of study and research on the cancer problem, the last 33 years in the U.S. National Cancer Institute, and with files of virtually all published literature on the use of amygdalin 'Laetrile' with reference to cancer, and with innumerable files of unpublished documents and letters, I have found no statements of demonstrated pharmacological harmfulness of amygdalin to human beings at any dosages recommended or employed by medical doctors in the United States or abroad."

But despite heavy evidence as to the complete safety factor of Laetrile, Krebs suffered a body blow in 1972 when two people on the West Coast of America were said to have suffered cyanide poisoning as a result of eating 30 apricot kernels. The story caused near panic to users of B-17 and B-15 across the United States. Apricot kernels disappeared from health food stores right across the country in the scare which followed.

It was shown that the couple ate a home-made brew of apricot fruit and stones left overnight in distilled water. The couple did, in fact, recover and it was never proved that it was the apricot kernels that caused the illness. The story, Laetrile supporters said, was purely propaganda to discredit the treatment. Certainly it got widespread publicity and achieved its results, if that was the case.

Wynn Westover, a young and highly qualified biologist and one of the leaders in the fight to legalise Laetrile explained: "If you hydrolise cyanide into free cyanide from meat, for example – just ordinary beef – what you do is to let it sit, mash it up a bit and put it in water for a couple of days. You would get enough cyanide out of that to experience cyanide toxicity. But who would normally put anything in water and then eat or drink it?"

I tested a large portion of Laetrile for myself – sprinkled liberally on a plate of ice-cream. It tasted bitter, of grated nuts, but I found it quite pleasant. Certainly I had no ill effects.

As Dr Dean Burk commented in a letter in 1972: "The facts are that a very considerable number of people eat ten to twenty apricot kernels throughout a day, and after a while even fifty to a hundred kernels safely, though hardly all at once as the . . . Angeleno gastronomes actually did. The same general situation holds with respect to a large number of ordinary foods that can be poisonous or allergic, etc., such as strawberries, onions, shrimps and so on, that are never removed en masse or in toto from food store shelves by health agencies imbued with the spirit of 1984 . . .

"It is one thing for a health agency to warn people against foolish and rare actions with respect to any aspect of health and quite another to deprive people totally of excellent food, quite safe if ingested in a normal commonsense way observed by 99.999% of the population."

When asked if it was possible to eat too many seeds containing B-17 and therefore poison yourself, Dr Krebs himself replied, "If we eat the seed with the whole fruit, it is impossible for us to get an excess of nitrilosides from the seeds. On the other hand, if we take apples, throw away all the fruit and collect half a cup of apple seeds and decide to eat that half cup of apple seeds, there is a possibility that we can suffer seriously from an overdose of cyanide.

"You cannot eat enough peaches or apricots, prunes, cherries or apples to get a sufficient amount of seeds to provide a toxic quantity of nitrilosides, but you can take a part of the plant and do so."

In other words, as in the action of Laetrile within the body, the fleshy part of the fruit provides sufficient rhodanese (protecting enzyme) to counteract the effects of too much cyanide from the seeds when in our stomachs.

When I went to see Dr Krebs at his home in San Francisco, I walked straight into the middle of the Laetrile drug smuggling row. The day I arrived, sixteen doctors and scientists, many of them friends of his, had been arrested on charges of alleged drug smuggling of Laetrile across the U.S. border from Mexico.

Perhaps ill-advisedly, the following day I set off on the next planned stage of my "youth trail" from Krebs' old world mansion, to drive by car to Tijuana, just over the Mexican border, where most of the illegal Laetrile supplies are manufactured en route to the U.S. I went there to see some of the main personalities in the affair to discuss other youth drugs with them.

But when I telephoned one contact from Tijuana's main street when I arrived, asking for directions to his office, the police were already there in the building. I was told not to come, and to call another day.

But who, I wondered, as I drove back across the border that day, in the U.S. Federal Police would have believed that I was innocent. That I had no connection with the smuggling rings and indeed, until the previous day, I had not even known of their existence.

But the real tragedy of the heartbreak route to Tijuana are the many cancer sufferers who travel down it to try and get the pills which they believe are their one and only lifeline. Hundreds of them, many of them terminal cases, often in severe pain, some exhausted by a trip of many hundreds of miles, regularly make the journey across the border by car to the clinics and factories where they can openly buy the drug. But on the way back, hanging on to what to them is their only hope of cheating death, they frequently find themselves searched and harassed by the Customs men, and have either to hand over the drug or are refused entry.

In the words of one patient, "Cancer victims are bullied, bossed, taunted and deliberately destroyed by those who should have the most care for them."

Another says, "My greatest fear is that they will take my Laetrile away from me and with it my life."

Wynn Westover says, "In 1973, I was collecting case histories and the Government seized my car, in which they found a notebook giving details of the patients. I was at the border at Ysidro. The names in the notebook were then followed up and patients were visited by pairs of agents who went into their houses and said, 'You're getting Laetrile. This stuff is no good. You are just killing youself, delaying proper treatment. You are paying too much for this material – it's smuggled material. Where do you get it? Who brings it to you?' and so on . . .

"They were then threatened with being taken to Court to testify about Laetrile. One patient, a prominent man, told me, 'I would rather die than have this kind of pressure. These agents walking into my house this way.' "

Meanwhile, the fight to legalise Laetrile has gone on. It is perhaps worth recalling again my earlier remarks that in the Hunza Valley of the high Himalayas on the Pakistan border, where apricots are the main staple diet of the people, sickness and cancer are not known.

Five years ago, many predicted that B-15 would one day begin to be accepted by orthodox medicine. Slowly this is beginning to happen around the world. Could the same be true of Krebs' Laetrile treatment? There are many, including leading scientists and doctors, who believe one day it will.

The most fervent believers are the cancer victims themselves, many thousands of whom say that it is thanks only to Krebs and Laetrile that they are still alive at all. The cost of a course of B-15 is around $95 (Australian) or just over $100/£50 and the cost of B-15 over the counter is around $9.95 in the U.S. for a bottle containing one hundred 50 mg tablets and £3.75 in Britain for 100 50 mg tablets.

Any queries about B-15 or B-17 can be sent to:
The McNaughton Foundation,
P.O. Box B17
San Ysidro,
California, U.S.A.
92073
or The Cantassium Co.,
    Larkhall Laboratories,
    225, Putney Bridge Road,
    London S.W.15.
    England.

CHAPTER SEVENTEEN

Plastic Surgery

"Prepare a face to meet the faces"

T.S. Eliott

Plastic surgery is the one sure way of turning back the clock IF you can afford it.

Nevertheless Hollywood's priciest and most successful plastic surgeon, Dr Steven Zax, sounds a word of warning for anyone thinking of embarking on it. "Of course we can turn back the clock just so long as people remember it will keep on ticking."

Steven Zax looks rather like a real life Dr Kildare. Ruggedly handsome, glamorous, he is, at only thirty-three, the epitome of everyone's idea of a top Hollywood plastic surgeon.

Our appointment was for 7pm at his home in North Beverley Drive, the heart of Hollywood's snobbiest film star belt of super homes. The trappings of success were all there as my taxi pulled into the horseshoe-shaped drive outside the long pillared portico of his Tudor-style mansion. It had belonged to Robert Taylor and Barbara Stanwyck back in the thirties.

The boyish young man in the open-necked shirt who opened the front door, grinned as I said I had come to see Dr Zax and waited with delight for my astonishment when I discovered that this was not his son, as I had imagined, but the eminent plastic surgeon himself.

He led me at once through the den, with its giant leather-topped bar, out through the old English gardens banked with roses to the terraced tennis court with its thickly tree screened tea pavilion. Leaning against the net as the warm, scented dusk gathered, the man, whose hands have shaped the faces of the stars, talked of what cosmetic surgery really means.

Dr Zax has a sensitivity and a sense of the aesthetic that puts plastic surgery, in his eyes, into the realms of an art form. "Good plastic surgery," he says, "should be a fine combination of technical adroitness, aesthetics and psychology. My feeling about plastic surgery is simply this. There is a wonderful amount of good it can do, it can accomplish things almost overnight that a psychiatrist cannot do in years of deep analysis. If it's my choice to do this, then I have an obligation to take care, not just of the person's breasts, not just their eyes, face or chin, but hopefully to impart to them some psychological, philosphical, emotional help also, somehow to influence them for the good, not for the bad."

But it is a path that can be fraught with perils if you are expecting that the surgeon's knife can provide all the answers to bringing back a lost love, repairing a broken marriage or simply set you on the road to an exciting new life. It may, if you are lucky, but don't make the mistake of thinking, as so many people do, that plastic surgery is purely a costly escape from emotional hang-ups. There's far more to it than that.

Considering cosmetic surgery has been around for so long, few of us know much about it. All of us know enough to have a cruel giggle over the ageing socialites who look as if their mouths are pulled almost to their ears and they can never shut their eyes. Few of us know the facts. Hollywood is as good a place as any to find out. Once upon a time the best plastic surgeons in the world were all reputed to be in Paris, Switzerland or Germany. Today the big league of professionals are playing in California. That's where the super ball is being held and at this moment it was right in Steven Zax's home court.

Film and television stars, we must remember, have always been ahead of the rest of us in using whatever beauty aids are available. After all, their face or body is their tool in carving out their art, very much like a carpenter would use his hammer or a sculptor his chisel.

Dr Zax speaks slowly, revealing an understanding of other people, rare in so young a doctor, as he delves deep and gently with enormous compassion into what makes people tick, what makes them strip their emotions bare and seek the help of the surgeon's knife. Hippocrates said once, "With holiness and purity I shall pass my life and practice my art."

"It's not always necessarily with holiness and purity," says Zax, "but people do want to practice their art and pass their life in the most general, kind way as possible for others."

The plastic surgeon potentially offers them one discipline, one avenue of hopefully continuing their ability whether it is as a star of a motion picture or television, or whether it is as a secretary, a housewife or a writer.

Everybody is basically alone, solitary and independent. You can have a gang of brothers and sisters, you can have a large family, but what it boils down to is how do you feel about yourself. What do I look like? What am I like? It's so hard to try and separate out what we look like and what we are. It is confusing not only to the patients but also to the plastic surgeon. There is something, after all, pretty scarey in facing a plastic surgeon, asking him to have a go at pushing around our eyes or chin, bobbing a bit off our nose, adding or subtracting a bit here or there to bosoms, tummies or even bottoms – to mention the most common trouble spots that drive thousands of patients a year to the plastic surgeon's door.

It is a pretty drastic step whichever way you look at it, whether you are aiming to preserve the good looks you think you have or are scared they are starting to fade or wrinkle, whether you know you are already losing them and want to get them back, or simply hope to improve on those with which nature unfortunately decided to endow you.

Dr Zax is pretty scathing in his view of many doctors who are today practicing cosmetic surgery around the world with only an ordinary medical degree and little or no expertise in the field to back up the name plate on their door. He says there are numerous doctors who see the way the plastic surgeon lives – wealthy, famous, making lots of money, living as well as his patients or better. Their own life style at the top, as perhaps an ear, nose or throat surgeon, compares poorly. Their whole medical training has in no way touched on the skills required by the plastic surgeon, but, by law, they can practice plastic surgery in many countries.

Take the *Los Angeles Times*. It is full every day of adverts touting for custom. *"Call now. Improve the appearance of your face, nose eyelids, ears, chin, neck,"* they scream in big print. *"Enlarge, reduce or lift breasts. Removal of excess skin from your stomach"*.

One doctor, who has had no surgical training but has a giant beauty clinic in California, claims he can augment or enlarge breasts in five minutes and have the stars back making their movie that same day. He invites them to come and have their face done, eyes de-bagged, nose bobbed and breasts made larger on Friday and have them back home on Sunday.

Zax says with disgust, "That's poppycock. You are in a position that is strangely unique. In a position where people are coming in and taking off their clothes for you. I don't just mean the clothes they wear. Emotional clothes too. They come in and you either covertly or openly say 'you must be honest with me'. And if they are not going to be honest with me, I pass."

"You mean you won't treat them?" I asked.

"That's right."

"Are there many people you've turned away?"

Dr Zax nodded, "Many."

Steven Zax treats some of the most famous people in the world. His consulting room is always packed with the faces that make the international news. His modern clinic in Century Park on the site of the old Twentieth Century Fox Film studios, has a side door through which the famous can slip discreetly; and a back door for when the press are watching the side door.

The waiting room is like no other doctor's waiting room in the world. Thickly carpeted in olive green, it has French antique furnishings, Chinese works of art, modern lithographs. The clinic is completely self-contained. Two operating rooms, three to four examination rooms, blue, green and yellow colour co-ordinated recovery rooms with even the paintings to match.

Beauty surrounds Steven Zax – his home, his wife, a former Miss Universe and the most beautiful woman, he says, he has ever seen, his children and the beautiful women, truly beautiful women, who flock to see him each day, Patients shower him with beautiful gifts too, Picassos, cars, objets d'art – he has received them all from grateful patients all over the world.

One of his patients, one of the three most photographed men in the world, is usually admitted personally through the back entrance by Dr Zax. On one particular day he came in alone and sat in the waiting room with everybody else until an agitated secretary spotted him and said, "Come in, come in – people will see you!"

"I don't care" he told the doctor. He was there with maybe twelve good looking women aged from eighteen to forty-eight. He said, "You know something? You have the best corner in town." What he meant was that he hadn't seen anywhere with quite so much exposure. There is no way in the world that any doctor, whether a top cardio-vascular surgeon or psychiatrist or a casting director could have quite so much exposure to more people of various bents, ilks or persuasions than Dr Zax.

Why is Dr Zax, and plastic surgeons like him, so successful? What has he got?

He cares. He cares about what is the right plastic surgery for his patients and he talks to them. It's no good going to Zax and asking for an Elizabeth Taylor nose, a Clark Gable chin, Bardot or Raquel Welch boobs – you won't get them. You will get what is right and subtle for you.

He says: "Everything should be done with subtlety and finesse. There is nothing worse than exaggerated plastic surgery. I have lots of patients who come here because they are unhappy, because they have been to a doctor who does the same procedure for everyone. It's a stock standard procedure and it's not appropriate for them. Their breasts are too large for their body or too small, or their nose is not right. It's important to be able to do nasal surgery so that it looks like that was the nose that should have been there before, not one that somebody's ego put on their face and it's too small, too pinched. or it's too high and you stare into the nostrils. You can walk down the street and say 'That's a nose by Dr A and that's one by Dr Q or Dr Y'."

One of Dr Zax's great successes is the subtle way in which he hides the scars. "It takes a great deal of work to hide the scars in the hairline or inside the ear rather than in front of the ear, and in the hairline at the back rather than running down the neck. I think it should be your prerogative to tell people whether or not you've had plastic surgery. If there's evidence from the procedure, it shouldn't be there," Dr Zax told me as he took yet another phone call from a grateful patient, many of whom, long after treatment, regard themselves as personal friends.

But who, when you think about it, can be closer than your plastic surgeon? After all, he's really carrying on the work where your parents left off.

If you think that the plastic surgeon is going to laugh or condemn your vanity, you haven't yet understood what he is about. Zax says, "I think it's hard for every woman although she denies it. She will say in a very apologetic voice, 'I'm so sorry – I don't mean to be so vain', and you try to explain to them that what they are feeling, what they are endeavouring to do is nothing more than the pride that drives them to bathing daily, brushing their teeth, keeping their hair and, hopefully, their clothes, clean.

"One patient was a mother, who is forty-four with a seven-year-old child and when she met him at school the teacher said 'Oh, is this your grandmother?' The first time it goes over the child's head and hurts the parent. The next time it starts them thinking. At that point they find themselves in the plastic surgeon's chair. It's a harsh moment of truth."

The girl bubbling behind the glass of champagne in the bar of Zax's mansion had IT. The look everyone else in the world is after. *The Californian Look.*

She was young, blonde, very beautiful, lightly tanned with smooth skin and sun-streaked hair, flashing white teeth and intelligent. Not only interesting and informed, but interested. She had also had plastic surgery and she didn't look a single day over twenty-five. She was, said Steven Zax, the ideal California girl and that, when it comes down to it, if you looked for the common denominator of what people are looking for in Mexico, Europe, Australia, New York and London, is the Californian. The Beach Boys had a song in '65 – *I Wish They All Could be California Girls.*

Why? Dr Zax sums it up simply in the way people feel. "There's a great mobility here. There's a great sense of freedom. Maybe what we are talking about when we are talking about beauty or the concept of it, is the concept of what it is that gives us the freedom. The freedom to be unafraid, to be secure, to be confident, to feel good, not just about what you do, but about yourself. If you are not going to feel good about yourself, no matter what you have done or what classes you take, no matter what plastic surgery you have, it's going to be to no avail."

Like all of the top, highly successful plastic surgeons, Steven Zax really believes in the importance of talking to his patients, understanding them and making them understand him. His attitude is that if people choose to come to him as a patient, he should treat them with the utmost care, gentleness and respect. "Perhaps you should give them more respect, more dignity and more gentleness than they either deserve or reflect back, but you will find that if you give them that, they will rise to the occasion. There is nothing lovelier than to spend the whole afternoon with patients who are just so happy and delighted that they are able to go out because of maybe what you have done or maybe what they think you've done. That's the trick – what they think you've done – and be able to function better because of it in every day life."

At what age do people seek plastic surgery? In Hollywood the attitude has vastly changed in the last decade. Once women waited until they were sixty-five and then rushed in hoping for a miracle that couldn't happen. Today, says Steven Zax, the youngest woman on whom he's done a facelift is twenty-eight. The previous week he did six facelifts, the youngest patient was thirty-eight, the oldest patient was forty-two.

Men are fewer in number but ten years ago 1 patient in every 100 was a man. Today, according to Dr. Zax, 1 out of 15-20 patients is a man. The average man will go in between thirty to fifty seeking help, mainly in his urgent desire to look younger and, usually, to have his eyes done or maybe a little under his neck removed. That's the spot that shows up age first in a man. Most of them don't need a facelift. They are much simpler to deal with and age is generally so much kinder to them.

Gay people, homosexuals in the main, go in to have their ears and chin done, said Zax: "It's strange, don't ask me why, I just know. But if somebody comes in at around thirty years-old and wants his ears and chin done you know that if you scratch at the surface at all you are going to dig up either a closet queen or somebody who is having a homosexual or bi-sexual life."

Much of his work involves putting right the botch-ups and bad work of other plastic surgeons. Take breast enlargements. Implants are expensive, about three hundred dollars. Dr Zax told me of one doctor who uses sponges bought from a local department store instead. This doctor, he said, wraps them in gladwrap, ties a string around them, makes a cut and shoves them under the patient's breast.

"I have taken out numerous pairs. If you have a bona fide breast implant it is as natural as the breast tissue itself; same motion, same mobility, specific gravity. It can be done so naturally that even another doctor cannot tell you have had an implant."

Dr Zax uses a silicone gel that is very soft and pliant. He puts it into a tiny incision maybe one half to an inch in length at the inferior border of the nipple just where it goes from dark to light. Within three to six months the scar becomes invisible.

"Previously I used to put the cut below. I did that for seven years but it was distressing because the scars were less than perfect and there was numbness because you were cutting a lot of nerves. Doing it this way you can augment, let's say, a section of the breast. The person has all the breast tissue that is demanded below the nipple.

"I had a girl here who had a breast tumor. She was twenty-one years old and it was the size of a chicken's egg." Doctors, who thought it a shame that she should lose a quarter or half of her breast, sent her to Dr Zax. "I made an incision an inch round her nipple and through that delivered the entire tumor. She could not believe it – nobody could believe it and everybody said it couldn't be done. When people say things can't be done it's very challenging and you think let's try and figure a way with a little imagination to do it and to do it better. She is just thrilled. She is so excited now. She is quite lovely and works for a well known T.V. producer.

Now she wants her nose done, her ears done and all these things. She doesn't really need anything done. She is just so sold on the idea that these things can be done this subtly."

The cost? Cosmetic surgery, any style, can be expensive. You can see from the pitfalls, however, that it is worth shopping around for the best and not wasting money on a botch-up which is probably going to cause you only heartache and more expense in the long run. Dr Zax is expensive. For his work you will pay anything between $1000-$5000/£500-£2500. On top of that, of course, it can cost you a further $30/£15 for an ambulance to take you home, around $50/£25 for a good hotel room and around $120/£60 for a registered nurse to take care of you for the first twenty-four hours. Their rates are usually $50/£25 for the first eight hours and half thereafter, but for this they will bathe the patient, cook for them, wheel them to the office and even take them out to Disneyland! If it is going to make your life all the better for living, it's cheap at any price so let's get down to the nitty gritty now.

The answers to all the questions every patient wants to ask from the right age to have a facelift to the chances of curing baldness. . .

CHAPTER EIGHTEEN

The Hard Facts

"Beauty is just a matter of a millimetre"
Phillip Lebon, FRCS, London.

The pavements outside Phillip Lebon's London consulting rooms should at least be glinting with gold. They're not. But his Silver Shadow Rolls Royce, purring fatly at the curbside, gives prospective patients the same sort of reassuring wink as they ring the doorbell and wait apprehensively for one of his curvacious secretaries to answer.

Mr Lebon is one of London's leading and most sought after cosmetic surgeons. He's also an expert on slimming and nutrition and has developed a revolutionary method of beating baldness by a flap method of rotating the scalp. On the first occasion I visited him, he had just concluded a phone call from a Japanese male film star offering to pay him $120,000/£60,000 for a top to toe plastic surgery job to make him look younger.

Even the unobservant couldn't fail to note the softly soothing air of padded opulence as they are shown into the ground floor drawing room of the double fronted mansion in Weymouth Street W1.

It is doubtful if many patients ever really take in the details – the deeply cushioned sofas, the deep pile wall to wall carpets and tightly drawn Venetian blinds. There's a colour television on the grand piano, and a few paintings on the walls – gifts from grateful patients.

The day I called it was hot with the stifling, stinking humidity of a London June heatwave. An old fashioned cool-air fan, wheezing and rattling its way round, provided the only relief from the heat, a stream of cool air for the man who had doggedly placed himself in its path, to the exclusion of all comers.

The few patients lying around waiting were either drowsing dowagers in pearls and shapeless linen dresses, who seemed too involved with their own problems to raise more than a perfunctory, unfriendly glance as I walked in. That's the point: almost everyone who goes so far as to seek plastic surgery is driven there by what seems to them an enormous problem. It may be only an imaginary line or wrinkle, so small that even the doctor can't see it – or it may be an ugly case of scarring or acne or an unfortunate nose that is turning their life into a misery and, consequently, the lives of those around them.

"But make no mistake," says Mr Lebon, "everyone who comes through this door comes in desperation."

My first meeting with him was little short of disaster. He was at the end of a typically long working day which usually starts in the operating theatre at around 8am and continues often until late in the evening. After keeping me waiting for well over an hour he led the way into his room on the other side of the wide hall of his clinic which stands only a scalpel's throw from world famous Harley Street.

Inside, his office is like a dark luxurious cavern. Black walls are relieved only by a few modern paintings, black sheer curtains drawn close over closed blinds. The only light around the giant polished director's desk comes in soft pools from large lamps shaped like huge synthetic boulders.

Mr Lebon wears American-style surgeon's garb of short sleeved white tunic, baggy cotton pants and white surgical sneakers. The nose is high and arched, the eyes pierce through you like a hawk. Who was I? Where were my credentials?

It looked as if the answers to the fifty questions which every man and woman seeking plastic surgery wants to know were to remain unanswered.

After a non-stop bawling out session, jet lagged and weary after my non stop travels, I ended up in tears and Mr Lebon, by way of a conciliatory gesture, said if I cared to phone him from Helskinki on my return from Russia two weeks hence we'd see . . .

A month later I returned to London and, with the aid of his glamorous wife, Pandora, who is in her forties but looks twenty-five, discovered during a three-evening interview a deeply compassionate man who understands the reasons that make so many of us dissatisfied with our bodies. Even if you never ever intend to have cosmetic surgery, reading his answers to my questions certainly leads to a greater understanding of how we, ourselves, and others feel about sex and ageing.

Here are Mr Lebon's informative answers on everything you could want to know about the A to Z of cosmetic surgery. As Lebon says: "The worst thing in the world you can do to a patient is to raise their hopes right up to the sky only to dash them to the floor afterwards." Here, then, is EXACTLY what you can expect.

Is cosmetic surgery appropriate for everyone?

What you have to establish with your patient is whether their aims, goals and objectives are realistic for themselves and their own self-confidence. That is my criteria for surgery. Will I, as a result of a surgical intervention, end up with a happier human being? If I think I will *then* I'll play their ball game with them.

There are two things I am interested in in my work – ageing and sex. That's what my work is all about. Your attractiveness, your body image, your appeal is a sexual thing or an ageing thing or both.

Every patient that comes to you is suffering fron non-acceptance of their body image. Otherwise they wouldn't come. Every person that crosses the threshold here is suffering from some form of inadequacy which they then project into some part of their anatomy. They might not like their nose, their face, their eyes, their breasts, their belly, anything about themselves. We do a lot of reconstructive work, too, after accidents, burns, etc.

But what we are practicing is surgical psychiatry. Take breasts, for example. There's a young girl who had a nice figure when she was eighteen or nineteen. She courts a fellow, gets married and has three or four babies. Her figure goes up and down, her breasts get bigger and then they sag or ptose and may atrophy. The psychological effects to her are of resentment: "I've done my stint, ruined my figure and now my old man's looking around . . ."

She's full of resentment, angry, jealous, everything. She comes to a plastic surgeon hoping he'll make her gorgeous breasts. That she'll have sex appeal again for her husband. She will have a reconciliation, patch up their life. She's full of expectations and she thinks that's what it's all about, while he's still knocking about with his bird on the side and probably hasn't cared a stuff about her breasts probably for three years.

The best plastic surgeon is the one who knows when NOT to use the knife. My criteria for surgery is after evaluating somebody properly, which means taking the whole case history, knowing everything about them, establishing proper records of somebody, really getting under the skin of the thing.

You already know, you have all the clues about them before they even get through the door, by the way they walk, the way they sit down, how tensed up they are, how relaxed they are or the way they look at you. It's all that body language before they even open their mouth. When you've got all that, taken the case history, I do a proper examination. At this point I'd like to get something right: all patients who present themselves for aesthetic plastic surgery have a different criteria or there are different perimeters of acceptability. Some people are looking for perfection not only one hundred per cent but one hundred and one per cent. Then I tell them they've come to the wrong address because nothing will ever be right for them. Somebody looking for this sort of perfection has the hallmark of neurosis.

But whatever the patients' problem I sit down to talk with them.

Someone coming in to get their nose done might expect a straight consultation: How much will it cost? When can we do it? How long will they have to wear a dressing? When can they go back to work? And then make a booking.

That's not the way to do it. You have to get to know the person. After all, I don't just sit any nose on any person that turns up.

The patients I've done work on you'll never know they ever had anything done to them. I'm always on the conservative side. You should always make an understatement of your work. You don't want to look as if you've had a face lift as you come out. What I want to produce for the patient is a predictable result. I want to be able to tell the patient, this is what I can do for you, that's all I can do for you. If you are asking me something else, I'm sorry, this is the material I have to work on. Don't ask me to produce something out of something which can't be done.

It's not good turning up with a picture of Elizabeth Taylor's nose, saying, "I want that nose," when they've got a plum pudding on their face. How the hell are you going to turn that into Elizabeth Taylor's nose? There's no way you can do it!

Do you do what the patient asks, or do you do more or something quite different?

A plastic surgeon tries to give what the patient wants if it is possible, unless the demand is quite outrageous or, for instance, totally out of proportion to the rest of the face or body so that he must try and convince the patient of this and come to some compromise that will look right.

Are people becoming increasingly worried about losing their youth?

Of course they are. We're in a very competitive world now and people are worried about being replaced by younger people who will do their job. And do their job better than them because they are getting slowed down and sluggish at it. Although they have the experience and the expertise they're getting older, and younger people are coming up so they're being jostled out of their position. How do they keep up with all this? They have to take some action if they want to do something about it otherwise they'll go under.

We live in an aggressive society – you must remember that – if you have a new born child it won't survive long without its mother. Its mother has to be there a long time, you have to fight for food, for water, for shelter, for everything under the sun before you can grow up to be an independent human being and provide all these things for yourself

The competitive situation is such that we have to stay as young as we can for as long as we can. Why not make available to yourself everything that 1979, 1989 or 2000 or whatever year you are in has to offer? I had a gentleman in about fifty-eight years old, but looking sixty-five, although he says he nips around, water-skiing, uses trick skis, jump skis, things like that – and he wanted a face lift. This guy is like Telly Savalas, shaves his head and has done every day for years. Now, how the hell do you do a face lift on a fellow when you can't even hide the lines of incision in the hairline?

Normally we would extend the incision behind the ear and across the hairline. In this case with modified lifting we can still achieve the objective the man desires. That is to take up the looseness and slackness of the skin due to ageing and the effects of gravity on the human body.

At what age do women/men seek the advice of a plastic surgeon?

The time when somebody comes to see you is when they want it – when they feel it necessary. What age they happen to be may not be relevant. They may be thirty-two and look fifty-two or only sixteen with lines around their eyes, through squinting in the sun, that makes them look like a sixty year-old woman.

Whether it is the right time to have the operation is a question they often ask, as they are worried it will be detrimental to them in future years when they really need a face lift. But if they feel they need it then the time is probably right for them.

Do some people come before they need a face lift?

Often people say, "I want that line removed." They point to a specific line on their face and you look as hard as you can, even put it under a microscope or magnifying glass and there's no line there at all. If they keep insisting, you've got to do something because they've come in desperation.

Do some people leave it too late before they come?

Take a lady of seventy-three years-old who comes into your office and says "I want a face lift. I want to look my best. I may live a day, I may live a year, fifteen years or twenty-five years, that's irrelevant. What I want is to look my best and I feel if I have a face lift done, then I would be very pleased and happy about it."

I think that's marvellous. As an example, an English lady, who has been living in California for a long time was visiting her children and grandchildren here – she had practically become a recluse and wouldn't go out or see anybody, mix socially or anything.

But when she was in England her children told me that she really wanted a face lift but was too embarrassed to ask anybody about it in case they thought her foolish.

This lady I operated on. She had a severely sun-damaged skin because she'd been living so long in California. However, I did her face and neck and the next thing I heard from her children was that she stayed in England another two or three months, she was up at the crack of dawn busy in the garden, gardening all day long. Before that she was just sitting in the house as miserable as sin and wouldn't even poke her head out of the door.

Is it possible to make a woman look twenty years younger than her actual age?
Simply – yes.

Where do the signs of time show first?
Around the eyes.

What can be done to improve ageing eyes?
The most usual operations are the removal of "hoods", sagging excess skin above the eyelids and the same below the eyes including "bags" or small pads of fatty tissues which herniate through the muscles.

The skin is also cut and smoothed out to remove "crows feet" or wrinkles. These may reappear with the constant activity of the muscles of facial expression.

The shadow in the groove of lines such as "frown" and "smile" can be removed by injecting silicone intradermically along the lines to fill the furrow.

Paralysis of the muscle around the eye keeping it closed or drooping can also be corrected surgically.

There are other operations including the "Europeanising" of oriental eyes and it is possible for eyes to appear larger by increasing the opening.

Do you usually advise a complete face lift or separate treatment, eg. nose, chin, eyes?

I prefer to do the whole job properly. I've heard of patients having the upper half of their face done because they couldn't afford the lower part. Then coming back for the lower part another time, the chin another time and the neck another time because this is the only way they think they can afford it, stage by stage.

I think any surgeon who's involved in the game is like a salesman involved in selling bits and pieces of a Meccano set, which means you can make only certain bits at a time, but the real bridge you want to build you can never make. I reckon you should save up until you can buy a proper Meccano set and build the bridge you originally wanted in the first place – otherwise you'll never have it.

Either do the job properly or don't attempt to do it at all.

Why does anyone need a face lift?

People often want to know the factors which make them look older, what happens to their skin and why they need a face lift? There are several factors.

The main cause is in the actual tissues of the skin: loss of elasticity, loss of elastic fibres, intrinsic elastic fibres in the skin, these become lost as the ageing process advances. Then the question of fat, the loss or gain of fat is very important especially around what we call the buckle or cheek areas. This either fills up the face or makes it look drawn and haggard.

Thirdly, there is the effect of gravity. If you see somebody lying down, for example, look at them again when sitting up. You will see the effect gravity has on the face in repose or in the relaxed situation. It's quite amazing and remarkable. You can wipe out a face lift just by lying a patient down flat!

How long will a face lift last?

What do you think I am – a gypsy with a crystal ball? I look in the crystal ball and map out the future for you. If you can fulfil all the factors we've been talking about, feed them into a computer and then programme the computer accordingly, maybe the computer will come back with the answer. Not whether or not you should

DO a face lift but how long it is going to last.

One surgeon I know in Paris, we call him Mac the Knife, incidentally, says: "Well, you are fifty-five, you are going to look thirty-five, so you'll be twenty years younger and it will last all your life because you're going to be that way the rest of your life after I've operated on you."

Although that sounds phoney it is also true. On the other hand, after a few years, depending on what happens to that person, they may need a revision of their primary face lift. However, one must ask about ageing in the family, climate, sun bathing, illness and overweight. Anything that will effect the elasticity and assess the type of skin. It also depends on what happens to the patient's health, and their attitude to their looks whether they have to be operated on again in the future.

Are doctors in general becoming more enlightened in helping patients to get plastic surgery?

There are lots of situations where patients are frightened to go to their doctors because they think he is only interested in them if they have got cancer or just had a coronary thrombosis or they are an interesting diabetic case or have some rare tumor. They see their doctor as a hard working, pressurised man looking after thousands and thousands of patients all day and all night long. And they think he will not be very receptive to somebody asking for help about a problem which is just vanity. You have to consider that vanity is a very healthy commodity.

A woman, who just came in to see me, had walked about in the same skirt and jumper for the last six years. She never went to the hairdresser to have her hair done. If I were her husband I'd want to know why she was behaving like that. Certainly I'd say, "Why don't you go out, darling, and get yourself a new dress or go to the beauty salon? What's the matter with you?" As it happens this woman came to me with bad acne scars requesting dermabrasion – she'd read something about it. She'd had bad acne in her late teens which went on to the age of twenty-seven. She's now thirty-five with two children. Her whole attitude was one of depression. She looked a miserable human being. When I asked about her past history, what illness and operations she'd had, it appeared that, because of some backache trouble, they took her appendix out and it was only later they discovered, after many X-rays, that she had a prolapsed womb.

When she went to her doctor about her acne he said something to the effect that she'd just have to live with it. He didn't seem interested. But she's only thirty-five years-old. She's got a premature menopausal hair loss on the frontal line of her forehead. I immediately put this lady on a course to boost her oestrogen level – she was getting old while she was still young. And, of course, she didn't like it. When she went to her doctor because she was worried about her hair loss he just said, "That's all right" – that's the sort of help she got.

In other words she might as well have gone to the post office and asked for some help. In the meantime she has now arranged to have surgery and I've promised her that her hair will greatly improve in the next six months.

Vanity is a very important thing. You clean your shoes in the morning, put on a fresh shirt, you see your finger nails are immaculate. You want to look your best because you want to present yourself as pleasingly as possible to other people as they should present themselves to you.

If you let it slide this is the first symptom that something is wrong and usually a depressive state. Depression is the overall result of unresolved anxiety, which the patient may not even be aware exists. Depression shows itself by the way a patient behaves, the way they dress, they way they walk, move, relate to other people and the way they relate to their family and anything else.

Why do you say that beauty is just a matter of a millimetre?
It's very true. It's a millimetre which makes all the difference. If you study any paintings, photography or look at the Mona Lisa, imagine the smile one millimetre away from where it actually is and you have got no Mona Lisa at all.

If you look at the statue of David, and there's not another statue like it in the whole world, it's a question of one millimetre which makes all the difference.

As I said, anybody who has had work done on them shouldn't look as if they had had an operation. But on the other hand if people don't say "I like your nose now," or "you've got beautiful breasts," or whatever it is, I might think my work is unnoticeable and therefore uneffective. But the biggest compliment I can receive from patients is when they have had plastic surgery done and not even their best friends or wives know, and they have got away with it because it isn't obvious.

The aesthetic surgeon's job is to enhance the beauty that exists in every human being, to make the best of what you have got – that's the message.

Is plastic surgery painful?

The question of pain is very interesting and here I have to talk about the threshold of pain. Some people have pain before you even think about it or look at them. They see blood and it hurts already. This is to do with the threshold. Some people can tolerate enormous amounts of what other people would call pain before they would even say they were in a state of discomfort. So it's very important to be aware what your patient's threshold of pain is.

Normally none of the procedures of cosmetic surgery should be painful at all. They may give the patient some discomfort afterwards but there are many post-operative drugs nowadays, if necessary.

I always explain to the patient what the whole text of the operation is and what they are involved with, because, for the patient, this is the event of their life. I know what they feel like sitting in the chair because I also have been a patient. But few cosmetic surgery procedures have much pain afterwards.

What is poly-surgery?

Remarkable things can be achieved, but sometimes a patient may want to indulge in poly-surgery, eg. after a sex change operation they might want a breast operation plus facial hair removed, nose and jaw line altering and a larynx operation for the voice etc.

All these can, but ought not, be done – other than the breast operation. The patient really needs psychiatric help to adjust to his new identity.

What has breast plastic surgery to offer?
There are four types of operation: augmentation: correction of ptosis (sagging): reduction: and correction of the ptosed breast with augmentation.

Is shyness a problem, for example, in the case of a woman who desperately wants to enlarge her breasts?
With enlightened patients and enlightened practitioners there are no difficulties, because the enlightened patient will not be shy, nervous or embarrassed to ask the general practitioner about the size of her breasts and neither will he be put out by it. If he is an enlightened person and he sees this as an emotional problem for her, or if she has an obsession or is inclined to be neurotic about it, he will understand the psychological implications.

A woman who has lost a good figure may feel sexually withdrawn. She may subsequently behave in a frigid manner and there will be overtones in the family relationship. Another reason a patient may be shy about consulting a doctor is that she is afraid the doctor/patient relationship is not confidential.

If you live in a small village or somewhere where everybody knows what is going on – even if you go to the doctor, the neighbours will know. "Oh, Mrs. Smith went to the doctor today. I wonder what's the matter with her?" and so on. Or you may be told, "I can't go to the doctor he's a great friend of my husband's," or "he belongs to the same golf club." All these things prevent the patient from enjoying a confidential doctor/patient relationship.

The whole family is subjected to increasing dosages of nudity in the media, especially in advertising and holiday brochures. Women are always reading articles about dieting and slimming, about beauty care and so on. The subject of plastic surgery keeps cropping up from a cosmetic or aesthetic point of view. After you have dealt with all the other features you are still left with the ageing body.

What can be done to reduce the breasts?

In principal you have to decrease the amount of breast tissue by incision of wedges. What you have to do is mobilise and then refashion the skin brassiere which supports the breasts. You must do it in such a way that your incisions leave as inconspicuous scars as possible.

Heavy or drooping breasts can be tightened, made firmer and lighter. Overdeveloped breasts can be reshaped. Before the operation, the surgeon examines the patient. Then, the first step is to measure up the breasts for a new skin brassiere. He marks out on the patient his design for realignment and the exact positioning of the nipples. After he has made his incision, the breast is lifted. Nipples and breasts are sutured in the new position. After two weeks the stitches are removed leaving breasts which are natural, but higher and firmer.

What about ptosis or sagging breasts?

It is important to diagnose, when a woman complains about her breasts, whether she's complaining of ptosed breasts or the size of her breasts. You diagnose this by looking at the level of the nipple, it should be half way between the elbow and shoulder.

It is no good augmenting a sagging breast because all you do is to make them top heavy and then they droop more. I solve it by refashioning the skin brassiere, if they have sufficient breast tissue – using incisions which will be as inconspicuous as possible. If, however, they have an empty, closed sac you have to use that plus a prosthesis under the breast tissue to augment it at the same time.

What can be done to enlarge breasts?

When a small breasted woman wants a better outline she usually envisages herself in anything up to a 36C cup bra. Before beginning the operation the surgeon examines the patient's chest in repose. Again he marks out the incision line following the grain of the skin so there will be no scars.

The extra circumference is produced by using a gel-filled sac or prosthesis which can be obtained in numerous sizes. To the touch it is as soft and natural as a normal woman's breast. The prosthesis slips easily into place beneath the nipple. Dressings are applied moulded to the new shape.

In an alternative method, an uninflated prosthesis is used clipped into position and then inflated with saline solution. At the end of the operation there is a curvy new look shape.

Is there a problem with cancer and breast plastic surgery?

What you have got to be careful about is that the prosthesis you are using does not interfere with diagnosis or treatment. There is no reported higher incidence of carcinoma in the breast in women who have had prostheses compared with women in general. I always say that at least if you've got a prosthesis in there, a cancer of the breast will probably be more easily noticed by palpation.

Is there ever a failure with these operations?

There is a subject of great controversy in the whole plastic surgery world – it is based on a post operative complication which is called "hard capsule". I believe that hard capsule is caused by small subclinical collections of serum, blood clots or many other factors. A subclinical haematoma is the basis of the pathology of hard capsule. So I believe in good, wide recesses to produce perfect haemostasis. For this reason my incision is usually a sulcus incision. If you make it in the right place you won't see a scar, or rarely.

Overweight? Is plastic surgery an answer?

Briefly, there are operations for the over-weight. The surgical removal of fat or joining the stomach to the colon. But these do not deal with the underlying problem. The causes should be dealt with, if possible, and the patient's weight kept down for a year or more and then an operation performed to take up the loose flesh and remodel the figure.

In looking at the body, we come into an area of sexual attractiveness in a physical sense, especially on account of the media. The general shape of the body is an inherited genetic control factor but it is also influenced very much by the environmental factors we live in, feeding of malnutrition.

People talk a lot about nutrition but not much about malnutrition. It doesn't necessarily mean we're starving. I think most people today are, in fact, in the state of malnutrition. They have too much fat and not enough muscle or vice versa. They are not balanced. They are unhealthy and if you look at their shape you'll see what I say is true.

Take a guy who goes for a yearly check-up to the doctors. He's about forty. He steps on the scales and says, "There you are, just like I was twenty years ago. What a fit man".

But the doctor gets out his tape measure and puts it round the guy's waist and chest and says "Maybe you're the same weight on the scales but as a matter of fact you are UNFIT." What has happened is that the man has lost his muscle and replaced it with fat around the abdomen. He is in a state of malnutrition.

White people, as distinct from coloured people, usually get fat around the hips and thighs and as they get older with their dieting efforts they get flabby inside the thighs and they complain about the bagginess and looseness of the skin around the upper leg area.

There are surgical manoeuvres to overcome this situation, some with quite a good success rate. Others leave bad scars and can cause iatrogenic disease in the patient. Personally I don't think there is any surgical treatment for obesity. The treatment is to treat the obesity!

What can be done for overlarged bellies, sagging bottoms?
Both these problems can be corrected surgically.

Is it necessary to keep weight strictly controlled thereafter, or does the operation have to be repeated?
The answer is that it is always important to keep the weight strictly controlled – but not by losing muscle and putting on fat and remaining the same weight as I described earlier. The operation, if it is correct in the first place, should never have to be repeated. If it's done properly once, that's enough.

If somebody comes to me with a big fat belly and says they want to do something surgically about it, I say: "OK, lose weight." They lose weight.

To me, the easiest thing in the world is to lose weight. The difficult thing is to keep the weight off that you have lost – in other words stay in control.

If a patient loses weight and demonstrates to you they can maintain the weight loss and then you repair their skin and you don't see them for five years and they come back as fat as ever again, weighing maybe ten or twenty kilos more than last time, then you have to start looking at that person's problems all over again, because it's probably a whole new problem causing the trouble.

I heard of a woman having her abdomen done three times, which means she got fat, and a bit was chopped off; she got fat again and they chopped another bit off; and then she repeated it all over again. I think all these operations were ridiculous, unnecessary and irresponsible on behalf of the patient, the surgeon and everybody involved.

This sort of plastic surgery is bad news. You have to get rid of people's bad habits and all the experiences that have gone before, before they can begin to avail themselves of what you have to offer them. You are bashing your head against a brick wall unless you have somebody who is receptive and cooperative.

Are there any psychological changes in patients after plastic surgery?

Yes. A lot of plastic surgery concerns physical signs of age. Competition from young people at work on the grounds of looks and not capability, or an inferiority complex caused by certain ugly features. Also it is a case of healthy vanity. If you feel you look good whether it is a question of a large nose or sagging jawline. Self-confidence can be found or regained through plastic surgery.

Can cosmetic plastic surgery be obtained in Britain under the National Health Service?

Most of this work is done privately and if the patient is insured a psychiatrically justifiable claim may be acceptable to lessen the cost involved.

The NHS will accommodate most of the aesthetic procedures with the sympathetic help of doctors and psychiatrists. But due to the fact that most plastic surgeons are already overworked, with congenital work and the results of accidents and burns, there is a long waiting list. It may stretch to four years or even ten years, which is no good if your problem is now.

The other problem is that under the NHS you won't know the surgeon who is operating on you. You may know whose supervision he is under but it will be in a large plastic surgery unit such as East Grinstead or Mount Vernon, or one of the plastic surgery units of the London Teaching Hospitals or in the provinces.

The point is, the relationship between the patient and surgeon will not be individual. In the case of aesthetic work it is an absolute necessity to have a first class relationship between the patient and surgeon, mainly because when a patient comes to you with an aesthetic problem it is a projection of an emotional problem through a particular piece of their anatomy.

The surgeon is the guy with the scalpel, but he must also be the person with great insight to determine whether or not he can use his scalpel, what he can do with it and whether it will benefit the patient. This is a very individual situation and my personal opinion is that I cannot see it being institutionalised like systems of the National Health Service.

How does America differ in its attitude to the plastic surgeon as a rejuvenator apart from the sort of work done after accidents, burns etc.?

In America everything becomes exaggerated, out of all proportion, particularly in plastic surgery. It has practically become a competitive field as though you are in the market-place and people shop around for plastic surgeons, compare prices and see where they can get it cheapest or who will sign their Blue Cross Shield forms.

In your view, can ageing be beautiful?

We don't lose anything by getting older. We gain. There are two ways of looking at the same question. You may lose what you think are your good looks but you gain in experience.

One evening, for example, we were dining with friends and they were discussing a certain lady's looks. What all of them overlooked was that different people bloom at different times in their life.

Some continental girls, for example, look beautiful, almost a woman at the age of twelve. At nineteen they can be way past their bloom, they've already lost the appeal of puberty.

This is quite common among middle-Eastern races. If you go into tribes in the jungle you find again their beauty varies according to the geography of the region.

I've noticed several woman who don't flourish until they marry and have children, and they may look their very best in middle age. Take Lady Antonia Fraser as a perfect example . . .

What is the cost of cosmetic surgery?

Ethically surgeons will not discuss fees and Mr Lebon did not discuss them. In London prices obviously vary considerably, but as a general guide: a complete face lift, usually a two to three hour operation, can cost around $1000/£500; de-bagging under the eyes from about $400/£200; and breast operations between $400/£200 and $8000/£4000.

Can anything be done about premature loss of hair?

There have been spectacular breakthroughs in work concerning balding and hair loss and this includes women, too. Due to many causes, women get thinning of the hair, perhaps they wore their hair in a ponytail or in a bun too tight for them for many years; or they might have had a face lift that left a bad scar; or loss of the sideburns.

All these situations in the scalp can be repaired in both sexes.

Why is hair transplanting not the ultimate answer?

Sometimes men get desperate about their hair situation and will literally clutch at any straw. That's why you've got all these different techniques of toupés and hair transplants; wigs, suction wigs, sew on wigs, hair grafts all with different labels, different sized packages, presented in a different way. They chop and change them about, call them by different names so that they will catch on and become more acceptable and commercialised.

These people, after all, are very vulnerable and susceptible to this kind of pressurisation.

Hair transplanting became available after it was tried half a century ago in Britain. The work was repeated in New York in the 1950's and it became fashionable after that. Showbiz got into it, everybody got in on the bandwagon and hair transplanting was on the map.

Now it's a bad commercial habit. The problem with this bad commercialisation is that we have to deal with raped scalps, unsuccessful operations. All many of the patients end up with, is a bunch of scars. The only really effective way of replacing hair is by transposing hair in a new rotation of the scalp technique.

What is flap rotation? Can it cure baldness?

The technique is a completely new breakthrough in treating baldness. I've been personally involved in it for almost five years now. It can have some spectacularly fantastic results. In my view it's the only really effective way of replacing hair.

What I'm talking about is transposing hair. In the technique which is called flap rotation you transpose in one operation eight to ten thousand hairs in one session, whereas in hair graft transplantation the maximum you could ever achieve would be up to five thousand hairs spaced over the total de-nuded area. With up to three flap rotations a man would get around twenty-seven thousand hairs to cover the same area. In addition, the patient doesn't have to worry about unsightly scabs forming around the follicle, hair falling out and a three month delay before regrowth is apparent as in transplants. With the flap technique, the hair can be placed where it is wanted, when it is wanted and just continue to grow.

How is the flap technique done?

It is usually a three stage operation. The first two stages are spaced at seven day intervals and can be done under local anaesthetic during an out-patient visit. The area to be rotated is punched out on the patient's scalp, usually from where the hair is growing thickly around the base or tonsure of the scalp. This is swivelled to be placed across the scalp where the hair is growing sparsely leaving bald patches.

The third stage requires a general anaesthetic and overnight surveillance. The patient will normally wear a bandage for five to seven days but could return to work after the second day if he wishes.

The hair which is rotated has been seen in dozens of cases to date to settle immediately and continue to grow thickly with none of the infection problems in normal transplants. The technique is not advised, however, for cases where patients are suffering with heart problems such as cardiovascular or blood dyscrasias.

CHAPTER NINETEEN

Hyperbaric Chambers – The Miracle Rejuvenator

The ideal candidate could be, "The vigorous executive in his early sixties, working ten hours a day – and who wants to keep what he's got."

Dr Eric P. Kindwall,
St. Luke's Hospital, Milwaukee.

Jules Verne dreamed up some amazing discoveries below the sea. But could it be, in fact, that in the depths of the ocean lie the answers which could solve many of the distressing problems of ageing and indeed of modern medicine?

Hyperbaric, or high pressure chambers are, or were until little more than ten years ago, used almost exclusively to help save deep sea divers with severe cases of the bends. Patients placed within the chamber are given a simulated "dive" which bombards the system with pure oxygen under pressure.

The techniques are still used in underwater medicine at many bases and diving schools wherever men go beneath the sea. But at the same time doctors all over the world started probing new potentials in the use of pressurised oxygen or HBO as it is more commonly known.

Fantastic, some say miraculous, results, started to appear in the treatment of many hitherto hopeless diseases. Heart attacks, gas gangrene, peritonitis, osteomyelitis, diabetes, strokes, cases of carbon monoxide poisoning, severe burns, and even spinal injuries, to mention but a few, all began to show amazing results. Time after time patients were snatched back from virtually the brink of death to start on the road to a comparatively speedy recovery.

Not surprisingly, therefore, hyperbaric medicine is now regarded by leading experts as one of the hottest and most helpful medical weapons in the fight against strokes, senility and the ageing syndrome.

It was, however, the discovery of some of its amazing side effects which put me on the trail of the men and women who live and work in the intriguing world of underwater medicine. Was it true, I wanted to know, that regular sessions in a hyperbaric chamber can greatly improve libido and increase the sex life of men well past their prime? Could it improve memory and cause I.Q. to leap in patients of all ages; retard signs of senility, improve skin tone and lessen sags and wrinkles?

Would it cause liver spots on ageing skin to fade, firm up breasts, turn greying hair dark again, improve nail growth and sharpen deteriorating eyesight?

There is vast and increasing medical evidence gathered from medical reports around the world to conclude that the answer to all these questions is almost certainly YES.

Yet they are side effects about which hyperbaric doctors are singularly loath to talk. Medical papers on their findings were not even published until as late as the end of 1972. Why? Because the medical researchers and pioneers, busy looking into what was to them the far more serious aspects of hyperbaric medicine, did not want their discoveries and, indeed, their credibility confused with what they regarded as the hoopla of the Fountain of Youth.

Yet time and time again, doctors in the U.S., Britain, Holland and the U.S.S.R., were coming up with similar side effects too frequently for them to be ignored. Finally, they were brought out into the open and discussed between curious doctors eager to swop experiences at medical conferences.

Now a number of doctors are eager to use the treatment as an executive "brush up" for men in their fifties and sixties. Indeed, a number of highly plushy hyperbaric clinics are already in operation – with more blossoming each year.

It would seem the potential is enormous. But, first, let's take a look at the background of this intriguing new treatment. Why has it been neglected, even ignored for so long when it has so many built in advantages which, it seems, not even the doctors themselves suspected?

The first medical use of hyperbaric pressure was in England when the British physician, Henshaw, tried the very first experiment as long ago as 1662. That was over one hundred years before even oxygen was discovered in 1771.

Yet as late as the end of the 1960s, tens of thousands of the world physicians and surgeons remained ignorant or perhaps just unimpressed with the work which was being carried out by teams of dedicated researchers in Europe and America.

Why it was so neglected is one of medicine's inexplicable mysteries. Doctors' traditional caution can be blamed but more likely is the wild over-exploitation of compressed air chambers way back in the dark and murky medical past of the mid-nineteenth century.

The French were among the first to popularise the idea, and the craze for compressed air baths became a fashion equivalent to the English flocking to take the health giving waters at spas like Harrogate or Bath.

By some strange quirk these early health doctors got on to the right idea and found that the saturation of the body with pressurised oxygen had definite beneficial effects. Patients emerging from the health tanks reported a feeling of well-being and by the 1870s the first portable operating tanks were being built.

The first was the brain child of a French physician, Dr J.A. Fontaine, who even had the vision to see his mobile tank being used in hospitals or wherever it was needed. How amazed he would have been to see his foresight coming to fruition one hundred years later with multi-thousand dollar chambers being installed in hospitals all over the world.

It was not until the early 1950s that serious work began again to establish clinically researched procedures on a technological level. The main pioneering work in this direction was done by a Dutch scientist, Professor Borema, and his colleagues at the Wilhelmina Hospital in Amsterdam in 1956. By 1959 he had managed to talk the hospital into building him a hyperbaric operating room and his first patient, a young girl, was an emergency case of gas gangrene. He put the girl in the pressurised oxygen theatre and saved her life. She was the first of scores of gangrene patients to be saved by hyperbaric treatment, many of them victims of the Vietnam war, whose cases otherwise would certainly have been fatal.

Borema's success stirred up interest, not only across Holland but also throughout Britain and the United States. There was only one problem in other doctors trying to emulate Borema's achievement. Few of them had a hyperbaric chamber.

At about the same time, a group of doctors, under the direction of Professor Illingworth, had established a large chamber to further their studies begun in 1955, at the Western Infirmary in Glasgow. Also in the early 1960s Professor Churchill Davidson of St. Thomas' Hospital, London, began preliminary work with hyperbaric oxygen combined with radiotherapy in the treatment of malignant tumours. While in the United States some of the first work was begun at the Boston Children's Medical Centre where doctors found themselves able to lease from nearby Harvard University what was thought to be the only tank in existence in America. The first hyperbaric surgery, however, in the United States was not undertaken until 1962.

But work across the globe was under way . . .

Popular world attention was first focussed on hyperbaric medicine through the tragic struggle for life of one very famous baby. That baby was Patrick Bouvier Kennedy, new born son of President John F. Kennedy. He was delivered by Caesarean section at the Otis Air Force Base, Connecticut, on August 9th 1963. But as the world's telegrams of congratulation started to flood in, his parents knew that the baby's chances were slim indeed.

Doctors watched in desperation as the tiny baby, weighing only 4lbs 10½ozs fought to draw in every gasping breath. But as each hour went by it became more and more obvious to the struggling doctors that he just wasn't going to make it. As a last ditch chance as the baby's little heart struggled to hold out against his heaving lungs, doctors thought of trying a hyperbaric pressure chamber. It had never been used in such a situation before, although it had been used successfully in helping to save hole-in-the-heart blue babies. Under the circumstances, however, anything was thought to be worth a try.

The dazed President, until now unaware of the desperation of the situation, was asked permission to transfer the child to Boston to the Children's Medical Centre where already the Havard compression tank was being made ready. He nodded his agreement and within minutes the emergency party was making its 67 mile dash by ambulance. Sadly, the baby was already on the verge of hyaline membrane disease, one the world's biggest killers of newborn infants. Nevertheless, the tank may have been sufficient to help give the relief he needed to his valiantly struggling heart to see him through the next few hours of crisis period.

The tank at Harvard was enormous. A giant boiler-like metal tank with glass portholes through which the President could watch progress. The hissing oxygen certainly helped at once with the baby's breathing but it was already too late. It was not enough to save him and at four minutes past four in the morning, when little Patrick Bouvier was only thirty-nine hours old, he died.

It was not marked down as failure for hyperbaric medicine – it would have needed a miracle indeed to save the child. But it was the first time that most people throughout the world had heard of a hyperbaric chamber – even if at that time, as indeed is still true today, they didn't recognise the importance of what they heard.

Today there are hyperbaric units in well over forty countries. Regional centres operate throughout the British Isles; the Soviet Ministry of Health has established a Department of Hyperbaric Medicine whose aim is to equip all the hospitals throughout the USSR with two or more single patient chambers – a programme which is already well under way. Programmes are already widespread throughout the United States, much of the research being spearheaded by the U.S. Navy at Long Beach, California, Japan has a huge scheme in operation and there are an increasing number of units being established all the time in hospitals and universities from Australia to Argentina and as far afield as Saudi Arabia.

What does treatment in a hyperbaric chamber involve? Originally hospitals went for large operating theatre type chambers which could take patients and a surgical team. This, however, was fraught with problems, not least of which being that everybody locked in the chamber had to be subjected to the same pressurisation, meaning that access to any of them in an emergency was impossible until the chamber was decompressed again. Otherwise they would have been subjected to the "bends" in the same way as a diver surfacing too fast!

Most treatments are carried out at two or, at the most, three atmospheric levels below sea level. This is technically referred to as 2 ATA or 3 ATA, and means simply that the atmospheric pressure is pumped up to two or three times greater than at normal sea level. The usual level used is 3 ATA, equivalent to a pressure of 2280 millimetres of mercury or what a diver would experience if he had plunged to a depth of sixty-six feet below the surface of the sea.

Therefore, patients take what is roughly the same as a deep sea dive – except they are not wearing an oxygen face mask and are, in fact, lying comfortably in bed. Sessions are usually for no longer than ninety to one hundred and twenty minutes at a time. The whole system is bombarded with 100% pure oxygen which, under pressure, is absorbed much more readily than under normal conditions.

In a normal human being breathing oxygen at 100% concentration only increases the partial oxygen pressure in the haemoglobin from 97-100% saturation, and the oxygen insolution of plasma from .3 to 1.9 millimetres per hundred. By increasing the pressure to 3 ATA, the oxygen in the plasma of the patient is increased by twenty times the normal; that is to greater than six millimetres per hundred which is sufficient to support all the body functions, including the brain and central nervous system without the content of the haemoglobin.

Amazing is not simply my word for results of hyperbaric medicine. It is one used by almost every one of the world's increasing number of enlightened doctors. They see patients of whose recovery they had despaired, beginning to respond almost before their very eyes. And all of them have been known to ask "Why, if this is so miraculous, haven't I heard about it before?"

It's a curious question and one that is not easily answered. Scientific scepticism or just plain apathy would seem to be the main solution put forward. Doctors seem to have been reluctant to talk for fear of over-exposing what would seem to be one of medicine's most vital new tools. Sadly, as a result, thousands of patients who could be saved by pressurisation are still needlessly dying each year.

In most cases treatment is usually given at the eleventh hour – as a last resort in an otherwise losing battle. Yet one can hear from those most closely involved – and those who are involved become almost totally dedicated to their cause – of new advances and new diseases that hyperbaric chambers are successfully curing or retarding, where before there was little or no hope at all. Each year, hundreds of operations are now being done in hyperbaric tanks. The problem in many emergencies is still that doctors do not know where the nearest tank is situated.

Take, for example, the killer carbon monoxide poisoning. It kills fast by asphyxiation blocking delivery of the vital oxygen to the brain. It kills hundreds of people every year and, even if found in time, can result in serious brain damage. Even if a victim is discovered alive and placed in the fresh air it takes over five hours of normal breathing before half the carbon monoxide is eliminated from the blood. Using the conventional recovery method, oxygen administered with a face mask at normal pressure, the time will be reduced to one hour twenty minutes.

But if the patient can be rushed to the nearest hyperbaric unit, the poison can be washed out of the victim's blood ten to twenty-five times faster even than with the oxygen mask. That means that at 3 ATA, using 100% oxygen, the patient's blood can be completely washed out in only twenty-three minutes!

Many would-be suicides and asphyxiated victims of fires, suffering from carbon monoxide poisoning, could be saved if they could be taken by rescue units to receive oxygenation in time. This is another vital reason why so many hospitals are anxious to set up units as a necessary part of their equipment, as accepted in everyday medicine as the blood bank, chest X-rays or heart units.

One of the world's finest carbon monoxide rescue stations today is the one run by Dr Eric Kindwall at St. Luke's Hospital, Milwaukee, who with his colleague, Dr Edgar End, was one of the first and most strident of America's hyperbaric pioneers.

Tank treatment is not always successful in treating strokes. But with two hundred thousand deaths per year in the U.S. alone from strokes, two-thirds of them under sixty-five, the method is regarded as an important breakthrough and certainly worth trying, even as a last resort.

As in all cases of heart infarction, the sooner the patient can be got to hospital the better the chances of recovery. In numerous cases of "first" strokes, patients have walked out of the chamber after only thirty minutes of treatment.

Dr End at Milwaukee County Emergency Hospital reports a case of a seventy-three year old man who had his third stroke in one year. The first kept him in hospital for three weeks, the second for three months. His chances did not look good. End decided to try hyperbaric treatment if it happened again.

Six hours after his third stroke the patient went into the chamber suffering from paralysis down one side and, although conscious, was unable to speak or understand what was going on. He walked, completely recovered, out of the chamber after thirty minutes and went home after treatment nine days later.

Stroke victims are usually given the equivalent of two dives a day. In Dr End's view, in cases of acute stroke, hyperbaric oxygen can be expected to minimise brain damage, reduce arteriospasm, encourage functional recovery and allow valuable time for doctors to diagnose and give further treatment. Most stroke victims, it is thought, given sufficient time, can recover.

Australian doctors at the Royal North Shore Hospital, Sydney have pioneered a world first using hyperbaric medicine to treat car accident victims with spinal injuries. By immersing the patient completely in pressurised oxygen they have saved a number of cases who would otherwise have been almost certain paraplegics as a result of their injuries. Doctors in America, also, have recently reported excellent results in the treatment of multiple sclerosis.

Some of the treatment's most startling results have been seen in cases of gas gangrene and in countries like Czechoslovakia, where today hyperbaric oxygenation is the treatment of choice.

In one of the most famous cases at the U.S. Naval Hospital at Long Beach, California, a young Marine was dying of grave shell wounds he had suffered as a gunner on the borders of North Vietnam. He was delivered to Long Beach, a mangled piece of humanity. He was badly ulcerated, suffering from chronic osteomyelitis, which is literally a rotting of the bones, and in addition he was partly paralysed and failing fast. After months of despair the doctors had to admit that the young patient was dying and there was no way they could help. Except for one doctor who absolutely refused to give up.

That man was Dr George B. Hart, Chief of Surgery, who is today one of the best known and outspoken names in hyperbaric medicine. Busily wading through medical papers for some sign of hope in finding a treatment, Hart came across a report from five British surgeons who had treated chronic osteomyelitis with hyperbaric oxygen. The result? Fantastic! Apparently the doctors had achieved a 75% cure rate. That was enough for Hart. He thought about the possibilities deeply and finally decided. It was a chance and he'd take it.

Waving aside the possibility that he would not get permission from superiors in Washington to borrow the Navy's nearby only decompression tank, used hitherto purely for divers, Hart went ahead assuming the responsibility himself.

To cut a long story short, the patient, now so weak he scarcely cared what they did to him, was moved into the nearby Navy Yard by ambulance. The tank was hardly one of the smart, gleaming modern units used today. But it would serve the same purpose. The patient was given a two hour dive, inhaling pure oxygen under 2 ATA. Hart waited anxiously outside. When the patient emerged he already looked brighter and pinker. Was it working? After four dives Hart had no doubts and nearly forty dives and much treatment later the young Marine walked out of hospital on his way home – cured.

There are an increasing number of new applications for the treatment all the time. Among some of the most widely used are in cases of severe burns and frost bite, gas gangrene, haemorrhage, heart disease, angina, arteriosclerosis, hepatitis, sleep disturbances and memory retention, stomach and duodenal ulcers, bronchial asthma, chronic bronchitis and slow healing post-operative wounds.

But for the man and woman in middle age wanting to hang on to the faculties of memory, youth and energy, which they already have, for the elderly, terrified of the first signs of senility and what it means, what has hyperbaric medicine to offer for them?

Senility, I.Q., The Sex Drive – Can it really help?
Somewhere, somehow we can accept that oxygen does play a key role in controlling the ageing process. So far, nobody has managed to unlock the door and put the pieces of this most fascinating of scientific puzzles together. But that therein lies the key is almost certain.

Oxygen, our cells, our brains – the question is what exactly adds up and how useful and energetic we can remain? Perhaps it makes sense of the indisputable fact that all the most famous of our long lived races, as I mentioned previously, the Caucasians, Ecuadorians, Hunzacuts and others, live in some of the world's highest and most mountainous regions with its rarified oxygen?

But the vitally important factor in the discoveries of hyperbaric oxygenation is that due to its magic we can be helped to remain mentally alert, looking and feeling more youthful and agile, and can retard that dreaded bugbear at the back of all our minds – senility.

At this very moment, millions of minds across the world are crippled by age. No news could be better news to the over-burdened medical services, sanatoria and hospitals caring for so many of them, than that in the future this heavy load can be lessened by keeping many of these people actively useful right into their old age.

There are now twenty-three million Americans over sixty-five, three million more than there were only seven years ago. By the year 2000 there will be thirty-one million and three decades after that these figures will have swelled to almost fifty-two million – more than twice the total now. In Britain there are more than eight million people over 65 – one in seven of the population. And if you add to that, comparable figures over the rest of the globe you can see the enormous problems the world is facing.

Just what do we know about the side effects of HBO, about which doctors so purposefully kept silent and indeed still prefer to do so? Dr Edgar End of Milwaukee was among the first to spill the beans but only when pressed with the question. Constantly subjected to hyper-oxygenation with his own patients, he had told close colleagues that he found that he had increased his libido. Although in his sixties and the father of one son and seven daughters, Dr End confided that he was as virile again as when he was twenty-five.

But he was not alone in his observations. Similar results were appearing in patients and doctors throughout the hyperbaric field. Mr Fred Jeffriess one of the world's leading biochemical engineers, specialising in hyperbaric medicine, has travelled thousands of miles each year installing single patient units for Vickers in over forty countries. He personally knows hundreds of doctors in his field, and confirms the reports. He agrees, however, that few of them like talking about this strange and unexpected aspect of their work. At the firm's laboratory in Basingstoke, England, Mr Jeffriess has collected together what he believes to the world's most complete library on hyperbaric medicine, including every available paper on hyperbaric medicine published so far.

So let's look at the evidence:

Dr Hart of the Long Beach Naval Hospital was, typically, one of the first to speak out. He was speaking at a lecture under the auspices of Vickers American distributors when he spoke of the case of a male patient who was having treatment in the tank for osteomyelitis of the jawbone. The patient was over sixty. However, only a few weeks after the man began his sessions, his wife came to see Hart. She wanted to know if she could have treatment too.

Hart was curious. Was there something wrong with her? Not exactly, said the wife. It was just that she couldn't keep up with her husband's sexual demands since he had been taking his dives. She told Hart that before it had been unusual for them to have sexual intercourse twice a year. Now – it was twice a week!

A seventy-two year old patient on hearing the story faked his records so that he, too, could get the benefits from an illicit course of treatment. He got away with five dives before he was discovered. There is no record of the results in his case, but patients everywhere have reported feeling suddenly restored.

One retired army colonel in his seventies had treatment and, only a few weeks later, amazed his doctors by marrying a woman in her thirties.

Animal studies using rats and rabbits have, of course, been undertaken, again with some convincing truth.

In humans, getting scientific evidence is slightly more difficult but it seems pretty conclusive that the hyperbaric treatment does indeed improve sexual performance. Among old men tested in senility studies, those receiving HBO had decidedly higher testosterone levels. Women showed similar results. The outspoken Dr. Hart again is quoted as reporting: "From my wife's aspect and my own aspect, plus my three secretaries who volunteered, the head of ENT, the head of oral surgery and their wives, we found that this does accentuate oestrogen and androgen output."

There is evidence to show that HBO can be of terrific benefit as an executive brush-up, and all round boost when the signs of age are causing them to flag. One seventy-five year old in Dallas, Texas, is a typical case in point. Like so many men past the normally accepted retirement age, he found his memory and concentration failing, his energy and vitality lacking, his limbs weakening. He came to hospital for treatment arriving in a wheel chair. After three or four days of two ninety minute dives per day, he was feeling decidedly better and by the time he left after two weeks treatment he was younger and more vigorous than he had been for years. He flew home and took full charge of his business again. The case is not isolated. There are many similar reports. The question of whether HBO can turn grey hair dark appears also to have much positive support.

End describes the case of a sixty-six year old physician who was partially paralysed by a stroke. Less than two months after starting HBO treatment he wrote thus: "After his third treatment he was able to overcome marked toe drop and raise his hands above his head. After his sixth treatment he was elated by the growth of strong dark hair into the margins of his bald spots. The cause of this re-growth is not clear. It probably represents an endocrine effect of the hyperbaric oxygen. It also resulted in a large number of previously reluctant and alopecic physicians suddenly volunteering to serve as controls by inhaling oxygen under pressure with their patients."

There is also evidence from many sources that HBO firms breasts and tautens the skin – improving the tone and therefore reducing wrinkles. Women who have had treatment say the result is the same over the whole body.

It is noticeable that doctors who have worked extensively on HBO do look considerably youthful and fresh faced. Coincidence? It seems not.

Vision, too, can certainly be improved in older people under treatment but the results do not last more than a few months.

One of the most intriguing questions of all is whether the treatment can, indeed, increase I.Q. as well as improving memory retention.

Again the signs seem to show that it can. Many studies are currently under way. Hart has once more been at the forefront, using himself and his wife as guinea pigs. At the start of the experiment, which involved a series of dives, Hart's normal I.Q. was measured. It was 132. After fifteen treatments it zoomed to 143 where it remained for nine months. After that period it resumed its normal level but after a further booster series with HBO up it went again.

For these reasons, doctors like Edgar End say they would like to see HBO used extensively as an "executive brush-up" treatment, ostensibly for people in their forties and fifties and perhaps even younger. He visualises this as a clinic treatment applied to high powered key executives. After all, he says, corporations insist on their top men taking annual physical check ups at places like the Mayo Clinic. But what they are really paying for is the men's brain power, their mental know how. He sees hyperbaric courses as the ideal for people under pressure: top government officials, scientists, politicians, diplomats and business tycoons.

Dr Edwin Boyle of the Miami Heart Institute is also thinking along these same lines. His main work is involved in reversing deterioration in seniles, but he can see the treatment being of great value to middle aged executives anxious to hang on to what they have for as long as they can.

One vital asset we all want to hang on to is our mental prowess. Previously the onset of senility, with its distressing memory loss and mental decline, was considered one of life's irreversible burdens. Today, it looks as if there *IS* an answer, certainly for many of us.

Take the typical case of this seventy year-old woman: all of us have experienced or known elderly people in this self-same condition. Seconds after having a conversation or sending her to do a small errand, she would have forgotten all about it. She didn't know her children or her grandchildren. She couldn't concentrate on the simplest tasks and would stand for ages holding a spoon or duster, trying to remember and simply crying.

This woman was lucky. Her husband was in the doctor's surgery when he saw an article on experiments being conducted on senility at the St. Barnabas's Hospital in Buffalo – the very town in which the family lived. The mother went into the hospital without much interest in herself, her condition or her future. She went on to the usual two dives daily for ninety minutes at 3 ATA, breathing in oxygen with a face mask.

Ten days later the patient suddenly started chatting quite normally, just like she had done two years earlier. With further treatment she continued to improve. She had become a person again. To her family, however short lived it might be – it was a miracle!

No wonder, then, that doctors like Edwin Boyle are anxious to see serious research continue as speedily as possible.

Meanwhile, there are many clinics already getting into the executive brush up business. In Fort Lauderdale, Florida, for example, patients can go and relax in plushy, thickly carpeted surroundings, while they lie back in the latest mobile transparent acrylic single cylinders and take their dives.

Today's cylinders are quite unlike the clumsy rather frightening metal earlier models and are now streamlined, gleaming luxury units. It's the cushy way to re-capturing the essence of youth.

Others advertising HBO purely as a rejuvenation treatment are operating in the South Pacific, Sao Paulo in Brazil and Lauderdale-by-the-Sea, Florida, (where it is combined most successfully with courses of cell therapy), Germany, Mexico and there are a number of clinics in other parts of the U.S.A.

Are they worth the effort and expense of having treatment? After talking to the doctors and engineers involved in many of them, I say they certainly are. But I do sound a serious word of warning. The results at present are transitory – lasting perhaps six to nine months before a new series of sessions is necessary.

But then, when you think about it, a session at the beauty parlour or the dentist doesn't last for ever either – does it?

The cost of hyperbaric treatment in the U.S.A is an average $75/£38 a session for clinical use. New clinics combining HBO with Cell Therapy are: Hyperbaric Oxygen Clinic, 925, Rua Henrique Martins, Sao Paulo, Brazil
and Ocean Hyperbaric Centre, 4001 Ocean Drive, Lauderdale-by-the-Sea, Florida, U.S.A.

Information on Hyperbaric medicine can be obtained by writing to the British Society of Hyperbaric Medicine, Hyperbaric Dept., Vickers Ltd., Priestly Road, Basingstoke, Hampshire, England.

CHAPTER TWENTY

How You Can Improve Your Sex Life; The Truth About Bio-Erectile Therapy And Penis Implants

"A survey shows that after bio-erectile treatment a seventy year-old man has a 58% chance of recovering his sexual vitality."

Ann Beveridge

There is no more sensitive subject than the problem of sexual impotence in both men and women, too. The sense of failure, frustration and misery is one which, all too unfortunately, the particular victim rarely wants to discuss with either their partner or advisers outside who *could* help.

Neither are sexual problems reserved for the middle aged or elderly. They can appear even in the very young, severely affecting the physical and mental ability of the individual.

And sexual problems, on the whole, are increasing, along with the stress that, sadly, is a bi-product of our era. Impotence is indeed on the increase in the Western world, particularly in Britain and the United States, and that doesn't only mean a man's inability to obtain an erection. It is a problem which goes much further. Of course, there are many men who just cannot obtain an erection which is distressing enough. But there are others where there is only a semi-erection which is immediately lost upon penetration or during intercourse. There are those who suffer from premature ejaculation, when the male ejaculates too quickly, often before insertion of the penis into the vagina, or delayed ejaculation when it is so difficult or takes such a long time the woman has long ago reached climax or lost interest, or where the ejaculation never happens at all.

Of course, few men will talk of this even to their closest friend or doctor – after all they regard it as a failure of their manhood. If only they knew how common their problem was – and that it *can* be helped.

In the woman sexual problems are equally common and distressing. For her the most frequent problem, of course, is frigidity, where she has a total lack of interest in sex or when the orgasm just never comes or is difficult. It can be a condition that comes upon her suddenly, or during a period of intense worry and stress, and then never seems to recover, much to her frustration and misery and, often, shame.

Another problem for the woman is delayed orgasm when it seems to take too long and her partner is too impatient to wait or help her along with perhaps physical or oral masturbation. Dryness of the vaginal canal can also result in painful intercourse causing frigidity or fear of penetration.

One of the greatest causes of sexual disturbances is the menopause or change of life – something that affects both men and women equally.

One hears little of the male menopause, but the man can experience just as many mental and physical changes regarding his prowess and capabilities in middle age as does a woman. Often he is putting on weight, worrying about his cholesterol level, his heart, his blood pressure and general lack of energy. Most of all he begins to concern himself over his attraction to the opposite sex as the obvious signs of ageing set in.

For the woman, of course, the menopause is something she has been prepared to accept since she first started the "curse" as her periods have come to be known since way back in her teens.

Many doctors believe that the early menopause is caused only by a set state of mind by a woman believing it will happen between her forties and fifties. Women, who have been unconcerned, have been known to continue menstruating into their nineties.

The usual symptoms, however, are distressing enough to the still attractive middle aged woman – today far more youthful looking than her counterpart of a few decades ago, due to today's better health, diet and skin care.

The most common signs of the onset of the menopause are well known: hot flushes, headaches, depression, flashes of unreasonable anger and irritability, sexual disinterest and dizzy spells. So what can science and the rejuvenators do for both sexes to avoid these most distressing signs of the physical division between youth and age?

Peter Stephan at his London Clinic has formulated a special bio-erectile therapy for men and a special RNA therapy using cells from the ovaries and anterior lobe of the pituitary gland for a women. While, also in London, is reported a new cure for the impotent male by penis implant.

Stephan explains his theory this way:

The formulation of Bio-Erectile M (masculine) is specific serums of testicles, penile tissue, nervous system, anterior pituitary gland and spinal marrow. Serums are obtained by injecting animals with specific cellular tissue of Bio-Erectile M. This in turn then reacts with the animal's own similar cells and produces antibodies to correspond with the injected cell material.

Blood is regularly taken from the animal and the level of antibodies produced is measured over a period of one to two months. When a specific level of anti-bodies is reached, blood is extracted from the animal and the serum is separated from the blood by centrifugal force.

Animals used for the process are kept under constant veterinary control and are maintained in a disease-free situation. The separated serum is then stabilised and each batch is then passed for analysis by the Swiss authorities in Berne before it can be released for general use.

Stephan says that two methods of application are used:
1. By suppository. The patient uses one suppository on alternate nights before going to sleep.
2. By intra-muscular injection every five to seven days.

The bio-erectile M. and F. anti-bodies then travel via the blood stream to the specific organs. How? In much the same way as I explained in cell therapy, it would seem that the work of transporting the cells to the corresponding organs is done by the phagocytes in the body. Radio-actively tagging the anti-bodies, according to Stephan, has shown that they travel only to the same organs as themselves and will not be found in any other part of the system. The bio-erectile anti-bodies, he says, attack the cells of the patient's organs which fight off invading anti-bodies. This causes a stress reaction which wakes up the cells and improves their function.

Unhealthy cells or diseased cells which cannot fight back are destroyed, leaving only healthy cells, thus improving the general function.

Bio-Erectile F contains specific serum of the ovaries, erectile tissue, nervous system, anterior pituitary lobe and liver.

In a survey of results of the male serum, carried out by an independent doctor, these were some of the results. The doctor defines total recovery as the ability to achieve and maintain an erection for at least ten to fifteen minutes and to achieve penetration and inter-vaginal orgasm at least once a week.

Case Histories

Company Director, age 65, married with twin boys. Gonorrhea during 1939 to 1945 war.

Raised blood pressure – not receiving treatment. Testes well-formed and firm. Normal up to age 61 – intercourse two to three times per week. Rapid loss of erectile power at 61 years.

G.P. diagnosed a psychological cause – no treatment offered. Two years later G.P. prescribed male hormone tablets – some improvement which disappeared when tablets stopped and not re-prescribed.

After treatment with Bio-Erectile M – after two weeks, erection improved. When re-assessed after treatment completed, could obtain erection at least once per week, hold it for twenty minutes and ejaculate inter-vaginally.

Widower, age 63, civil engineer and surveyor, four children.

No medical abnormality detected. Blood pressure normal,

testes well formed and firm. Frequency of intercourse when normal was two to three times a week. Noticed waning sexual powers at age 59, gradually worsening until complete impotency ten months ago.

After treatment – now obtaining good erection and ejaculation.

Retired writer, aged 61, married twice, two children.

No medical abnormality. Testes soft and small, blood pressure normal.

Sexual history normal up to age 58, one year after marriage to younger woman. Intercourse to orgasm average once a week. Difficulty in past three years – loss of penile sensation – erection less firm – able to penetrate but not ejaculate.

After treatment – by end of treatment erection firm and now able to ejaculate at least once a week. Spontaneous early morning erection has returned together with increased sensation and response to sexual stimulation.

Company Director, age 58, married, three children.

Medical history: coronary thrombosis 1971 – good recovery. Testes well-formed and firm. Blood pressure normal.

Sexual history showed twenty years difficulty in obtaining and holding erection. Hormone therapy failed to improve condition. Complete impotence for last three months.

After treatment: restored potency. Firm erection lasting thirty minutes if necessary to achieve wife's orgasm – then able to have own ejaculation. Feels much more confident in every respect.

Teacher, age 52, married.

Medical history: suffered from insomnia for which he took Mogaden. Clinical examination showed no abnormality, testes normal size but soft. Blood pressure normal. Sexual history showed intermittent attacks of impotency and at time of interview had been impotent for three months.

After treatment: return to normal with good erection and intervaginal ejaculation. In addition his sleep rhythm had returned to normal – he had stopped taking sleeping tablets.

Plumber, aged 52, married with three children.

Clinical examination showed raised blood pressure but no symptoms. Testes well-formed and firm. Sexual history showed period of semi-impotence at age 40 to 44. He then recovered but for the past two years had experienced return of failure to obtain or sustain erection and consequently no inter-vaginal penetration. Had stopped all attempts at sexual intercourse nor did he masturbate having lost all his desire.

After treatment had experienced full return of his libido, making him feel younger with increased drive in all areas of his life. Erections are now full and he is able to achieve inter-vaginal orgasms three times a week.

The survey included 103 volunteers each of whom was given a course of either six intra-muscular weekly injections of Bio-Erectile or six weeks treatment with Bio-Erectile suppositories. Of the 103 patients, 93 completed the course and 89 were assessed, 64 of these between the ages of 40 and 60. The result of the survey showed an overall improvement in sexual response among the volunteers of 77.5% and a total recovery rate of 59.5%.

According to these figures, a male of up to seventy years of age has the possibility of a 58% minimum chance of recovering his sexual vitality towards an improved sex life.

There have been many weird and wonderful ways tried in the last few years to boost up the impotent male with ideas like artifical implants, hollow dildos and even splints, which haven't been exactly popular with the sufferer's female partner, often causing extreme pain in use. However, the increasing number of impotent patients has resulted in doctors and scientists pushing ahead with their researches for a successful answer to this very root of man's virility.

Impotence is, of course, not always caused by psychological problems. Often men become afflicted as a result of accidents, car crashes or nervous disorders in addition to diseases like diabetes, kidney failure, complications of prostrate surgery, drug therapy or illnesses like arteriosclerosis, so much more common now in advancing age.

However, hope is now at hand by a new method of penis implant being carried out privately by surgeons in London. A patient can probably be helped back to full sexual function by a new and simple operation – having a small carrion penile prosthesis implanted into his penis. The result gives the patient a permanent semi-erection, but most men are so delighted by their new vigour that the slight manly bulge in the pubic area is usually a cause for delight rather than embarrassment!

The operation is comparatively simple, as I have said. The penis has two sets of muscles, both hollow, called the corpora cavernosa which, in the past, have been opened and filled with artificial stiffeners – without much success.

The new small-carrion prostheses are made from a gel inserted inside two bi-lateral rods, each filled with a stabilising layer of sponge. The rods are firm but flexible enough to be comfortable and are sufficiently far back into the groin to provide a secure basis for erection. The rods are curved but thin towards the ends nearest the groin to avoid discomfort and, in effect, provide a simulated penis bone. The operation cannot, of course, increase the natural length of the penis.

In order to put the implants in place, the surgeon will make a vertical incision an inch and a half long at the base of the penis near the perineum. He next inserts two dilators to open out the two sets of muscles so that he can insert the prostheses. These fit on either side of the penis, the curved ends tucked neatly back into the muscles of the groin.

The operation is performed, of course, under general anaesthetic and the patient usually stays in the clinic for two to three days afterwards for observation to make sure that healing is normal and urination painless and uncomplicated. Complete healing takes about a fortnight and the patient can undertake intercourse within two to three weeks.

As I have mentioned earlier, sexual potency in both men and women can be much improved by undergoing cell therapy treatment, which has been seen to restore sexual vigour quickly in both sexes. Also, Ana Aslan claims that her Procaine treatment, Gerovital H3, as well as KH3 pills, helps considerably in restoring a satisfactory sex life.

Hyperbaric HBO treatment, as I described earlier, is without doubt one of the fastest ways of restoring libido as doctors working in the chambers have been the first to report. The failure to enjoy a happy and satisfactory sex life is not a problem that has to be accepted as one of the sad losses of old age. If you have the will to do something about it – there is a way!

CHAPTER TWENTY-ONE

The Millionaire Clinic In The Bavarian Alps.
The Secret Of Bogomoletz Serum

"We can make the skin and glands younger and we can give more vitality and health."

Dr Fritz Wiedemann

Fritz Wiedemann was among the first of the modern day rejuvenators to climb on to the get-rich bandwagon by opening a luxury youth clinic, claiming he could retard age by a good 10-12 years, and coined himself in the process a cool fortune. Today, the wealthy Wiedemann, a bespectacled Munich neurologist, lives with his family in a two-wing villa overlooking the real-life Peter Pan paradise he created.

Anyone who doubts the existence of the whole keep-young merry-go-round, the eagerness of Mr and Mrs Average, as well as the rich, to roll up in their thousands for a chance of cheating the passing years, should take a look, as I did, at Sanatorium Wiedemann. It is one of the most amazing clinics of its kind in the world.

All the way across Europe my curiosity grew. Not just in Dr Wiedemann and his money-spinning ventures – he has four clinics today strung across Germany – but in the main treatment he uses called Bogomoletz serum. Discovered originally by a Russian, the late Professor A. A. Bogomoletz in Kiev, it has now been developed by Wiedemann and forms the main basis of his rejuvenation treatment. And everywhere I went to visit laboratories and doctors I repeatedly heard about the amazing "Mr Five Per Cent of Munich" – the nickname with which they have tagged Wiedemann for the way in which he so successfully sells his treatments around the world under licence to other youth doctors and their clinics. His methods are being used by 800 medical pratitioners in Germany alone.

By the time I reached Berlin there was no question in my mind as to where I was heading next. Ambach was just an insignificant dot on the map of Southern Europe, a tiny village in the foothills of the Bavarian Alps, situated on the shores of the tranquil and beautiful Starnberger See. So it was on that hot, sunny day I found myself travelling by taxi through the country lanes, between the tall grass of fields and hedgerows filled with summer flowers, and the sound of gently tinkling bells as the gentle, pale cows with their soft, fringed eyes turned curiously to watch me pass.

A quick turn up a steep grassy incline and we were there. A carved Bavarian sign on an old stone wall, tumbled about with blossoms, announced gravely, Sanatorium Wiedemann.

But even the surprising world of the whole rejuvenation scene had left me unprepared for this. It was exactly like stepping into a Hollywood film set – this spot, which attracts well over 6000 tourists every year, many of them Americans on package tours to Europe, looking for youth and better health as their holiday bonus. The attractive German receptionist in the cool, round entrance hall appraised me politely and, pointing me down the path, sent me off in the direction of Dr Wiedemann's private home.

I found myself looking down on a flower-filled valley where time really did seem to be standing still. People, mainly elderly, were moving gently back and fro like automatons in straw hats. Elderly blondes, fat dowagers, balding men in Tyrolean hats and here and there a young woman – intent, perhaps, on staving off the wrinkles before they began?

As I descended the path, I was struck by the unreality of the scene. The sculptured landscape of almost idyllic beauty, the terraces with their rashes of bright striped umbrellas, the film star pool with its stained glass windows and silken rope surround, the graceful villas each converted into rooms in a different style, the sparkling waters of the lake below and the over all silence, the sense of tranquility and peace.

I wandered slowly down the path looking at the guests I passed.

The illusion was complete. Glamorously dressed, each looked exactly like a tourist at a luxury hotel. Yet I knew, and they each knew, they were all here for a purpose – for the daily visit to the modern buildings hidden from sight at the bottom of a steep slope, the Kur Praxis or Clinic, where a team of doctors, each armed with a syringe, could *perhaps* make their dreams come true.

As I entered the Clinic building the morning session was in full swing. Guests, trying not to look at each other, were sitting expectantly waiting their turn while a queue of newcomers lined up at the desk waiting for appointments for their check-up and medical.

"Dr Wiedemann?"

"No, round the corner," the girl directed me onward to the beautiful villa on the outskirts of the enormous grounds.

The whole complex is run completely by the Wiedemann family – the clinic by Fritz and the hotel side by his son, Herr Helmut Wiedemann, who lives in one wing of the villa.

Wiedemann, himself, was surprising for such an enterprising tycoon as well as a prolific researcher and writer. He is small, shy, quiet, almost retiring with huge, thick, pebbled glasses and a gentle smile. People write to him from all over the world as Fritz Wiedemann, "the Kur Home, Bavarian Alps, West Germany" – and it finds him.

The clinic takes about 400 patients at one time. They come in the main, Dr Wiedemann explained, for a three week stay. There is a shorter ten-day treatment for holidaymakers in a hurry, although the three-week course is recommended for the best results.

Dr Wiedemann describes his treatment as "biological regenerative therapy," and, like most youth doctors, dislikes the word "rejuvenation". About 50% of his treatment is basic rejuvenation for the whole body, he says, the rest is for specific illness or problems.

According to Dr Wiedemann, regeneration from his treatment can lengthen the biological age of the patient by 10–20 years; it can turn grey or white hair darker and, in 80% of cases, the skin loses its age lines. Many of his patients, however, come to him with specific illnesses, such as heart disease and arthritis, headaches and stomach disorders and much of his work nowadays is also devoted to the treatment of backward children.

One 81 year-old woman patient who, Dr Wieldemann says, was crippled with arthritis when she first came to the clinic, could, two years later, go for a three-hour walk every day and her biological age improved to "about sixty."

Dr Wiedemann began his series of treatments originally by developing the Bogomoletz serum, which is said to have originated during researches to find a rejuvenation treatment for Stalin.

Bogomoletz maintained that the ageing process is connected with the mesemchyme or connective tissue of the body, which exists all over the human body. He found he could stimulate this tissue by injecting his serum, obtained from the spleen and bone marrow of young, fatal accident victims. This was then injected into laboratory rabbits, creating antibodies, and the resulting anti-reticulum cytotoxique serum could then be reinjected back into the connective tissue resulting in regenerative stimulation – a younger looking and younger feeling human being.

Taking this as the basis, over the last twenty years Dr Wiedemann has developed twelve different sera as treatment for many illnesses and for almost every organ of the body. He claims he can certainly make some patients look twenty years younger than their calendar age.

"We can make the skin and the glands younger, sometimes the organs, but certainly we can give more vitality and health. And if you are healthy you feel better and look younger."

The Ambach Clinic also has a Department of Psychiatry for Nervous Problems and, as well as the various sera, includes a number of other rejuvenation treatments. They include Regeneresen – the brand of cell therapy using RNA and DNA, synthesised protein; Schwarzhaupt, Municaps, a booster Procaine treatment in capsule form; Dimethylaminoaethanol (D.M.A.E.); and a new development, which Dr Wiedemann calls H7.

His philosophy seems to be "the more the merrier" on the theory that one of the treatments is bound to do some good. The treatment doesn't only consist of the injections. The whole life-style at the centre is aimed at restoring the human body to health –

and in many ways like the popular "health farm".

The diet during a patient's stay is packed with protein with very few carbohydrates and contains no alcohol, no tea and no coffee at all. Guests drink peppermint, camomile and rose-hip tea or fruit juices, and there are two "dry" days a week.

The calorific content is between 1600 and 2000 calories a day. If you take a specific slimming cure during your stay this is cut to 800 calories a day. No wonder guests go home an average eight pounds lighter than when they arrive!

Wiedemann doesn't lay any claims to the length of time "Die Kur" will last but he does recommend people should return for a booster or refresher every two years. The majority of people who go to Ambach for treatment are between the ages of 40 and 60, women starting at about 40 and men 15 years later, but these days many more are going from the younger age brackets. Many of the patients at Ambach are, in fact, from the medical profession themselves.

Dr Wiedemann heads a team of ten doctors at his Kur Praxis who carry out the initial medical and he will then see each patient nine times for injections during a three-week stay. Injections are usually given in the morning every other day, leaving guests free to enjoy their holiday or rest in between, as they will.

Most of the people I spoke to at the Centre were enthusiastic about the treatment and their hopes of a cure. Many had travelled from as far afield as America, South Africa and Brazil.

Clearly, I cannot vouch for the authenticity of Wiedemann's treatment. I can only tell you that many clients return again and again but with such an idyllic holiday spot as Ambach and Starnberger Lake, who wouldn't – for the holiday facilities alone?

I must admit I was surprised at the comparatively low cost for such millionaire-style surroundings. There are nine separate buildings and a choice of rooms, ranging from the super luxury bracket to comfortable, typical Bavarian style – all beautifully furnished, spotlessly clean and carefully maintained by the fifty-strong staff.

Facilities include massage rooms, ozone sauna, games and television rooms and individual sitting rooms in each of the villas to change your view and surroundings with your mood. The restaurant, with its shiny blue ceramic floor has huge, modern, mirrored windows, while the reception lounge is sheer splendour with deep pale turquoise velvet chairs in their wood and brass frames, and a circular bar and seating area in which to sip non-alcoholic drinks.

Around the Centre are some of the most beautiful walking areas in the world and the lake is stacked with good fishing, pike, eel and perch, for which the visitor can get a local fishing permit for his or her stay. And there's yatching, boating and tennis and golf, too, for the energetic get-fit addict.

For this the cost is DM1100-DM1500 ($579-$790/£282-£385) per 2/3 week treatment including medicines, and the price for the room with full board ranges from DM90-DM130 ($47-$68/£23-£33) per day. There are extra charges for special treatments, say for arthritis or heart trouble but basically you could expect to pay about $200/£100 for a three-week course of treatment plus board. My view is that the Sanatorium Wiedemann gives good value for money. The address is: Sanatorium Wiedemann, Ambach am Starnberger See, Bavarian Alps, West Germany. It is almost one hour's drive by road from Munich International Airport.

CHAPTER TWENTY-TWO

Back To Youth — Inch By Inch

"My personal opinion is that obesity is a disease entity in its own right."

Phillip Lebon,
M.B., B.S., M.R.C.S., L.C.P., F.R.C.S. (Ed.)
Vice President of the Obesity Association.

Most of us at sometime in our lives have waged a silent and often losing battle against the weighing scales and the calories in an effort to become a slimmer version of ourselves. Unfortunately, food and drink are among the greatest enjoyments for most human beings, but today there can be few of us who are left unaware of the important connections between good and balanced nutrition and good health.

This is not a book on slimming — indeed there are many thousands of other expert editions on the market to cope exclusively with the subject. However, what we are concerned with is health in relation to extending our life span, as well as looking younger, and there is a very close connection between obesity and gerontology.

It is a known fact and statistically proven that people who are obese are reducing their life expectancy. Figures available today show that being even ten pounds overweight will reduce the normal life expectancy of a person by 8%; twenty pounds by about 25% and thirty pounds by maybe 40%; fifty pounds by more than 50%. Therefore, if you carry around a large amount of excess weight you are not even giving yourself the same chance as if you sat down at a roulette table. Furthermore, overweight is associated with lack of activity and, therefore, a consequent lack of fitness. By keeping a slim figure and trim body one normally tends to do at least some exercise as well, and the combination of the two, normal body weight plus good muscle tone, will certainly be conducive to a longer, healthier life.

First, let us take a look at what obesity is and its causes, and then some of the more scientific methods that are being evolved by doctors, in addition to diet, in order to alleviate it and help us to control our bad eating habits.

The trouble is that most of us are loath to admit that our fatness is caused by our own abuse of nutrition. How often does the patient, facing the doctor for the first time, insist that "there is something wrong with my glands."

Unfortunately, even today medical schools teach little about obesity as a disease entity in itself. Only recently has sufficient – and still pitifully little – attention been paid to the importance of nutrition in preventing disease as well as curing it.

Phillip Lebon, a London Harley Street slimming consultant and plastic surgeon, who has long been involved in the problems of obesity, believes that it is a disease in its own right.

Apart from the few diseases of which it is a complication, the busy doctor confronted by his overweight patient often becomes involved in helping the patient to shift the blame away from their own guilt. In this he denounces the most common excuses expounded within the surgery "Bonny bouncing babies, puppy fat, middle aged spread, eating for two when pregnant, feeding a cold and the rest . . ."

All the patient really wants to know is "What do I do about my overweight?" Instead the overworked practitioner, running around overloaded with chores, confronted with crises every hour, takes the easy way out. After all, he usually reasons, obesity is not a problem that requires an immediate solution, he does not have an immediate solution and he'll dismiss the whole matter with sympathetic clucking and the remark, "You'll have to go on a diet and eat less."

The patient will leave with the latest diet sheet in his hand and perhaps, if he is lucky, a sample of the newest anorexiant drug, which a generous rep happened to leave with the doctor on his last visit and which merely has the effect of pepping you up and making you less aware of your mental hunger.

The important factor to recognise is that it is this mental hunger, when you eat over and above your physical requirements, when you eat with your eyes, when you eat with your mind, when you eat out of boredom, spite or misery – and not just physical hunger, that is the main cause of obesity. Very seldom do you find an undomesticated animal who will eat unless it is hungry. Even a new born pup cannot be forced to eat. Certainly not a new born child. You have to educate them to accept the amount of food you force down their throat.

If you left it to children to express their normal desires of hunger you would only feed them when they were crying and they would only cry when they were hungry unless there was some other physical cause. We educate our children from early childhood to adopt the eating habits of our particular race, which we have acquired, correctly or incorrectly, over the years – usually more wrongly than rightly. That is why the children of fat parents are generally fat – and the same of thin parents. It is not an hereditary condition but our eating habits that are hereditary.

Going back to the use of anorexiants – they are only a crutch. They will suppress the hunger temporarily but will not solve the cause of it. They tend to be addictive and, for this reason, are not prescribed by many doctors these days. In the same way, some doctors give patients diuretics – an agent that will help remove excess fluid from the body. They are widely used in health farms for showing dramatic weight loss on the scales but they are only removing fluid. It's a self-delusion for the patient who is losing only water – not fat – since water is even heavier than fat. One pound of water will be equal to less than a pound of fat.

As Dr Pawan, a consultant on nutrition and obesity at London's Middlesex Hospital points out: "You can give people anorectic agents, diet sheets and any amount of prescriptions, but in the long run it is the person who has to deal with the problem. No amount of talking from the doctor is going to make them slim. It is mainly the ideological factor. No doubt there are some people who fatten easily. But one of the problems as we get older – past 50 – we tend to lose lean tissue and replace it with fat tissue. The percentage of fat goes up and the tissue goes down although your weight may not change. One of the effects of ageing, also, is to reduce your metabolic rate and if you still maintain the eating pattern you had when younger and more active, obviously you will be taking more calories than you require and the result is you tend to get fatter.''

The sad fact is that so few doctors have a thorough understanding of the problems of obesity, despite the fact that it is so vital to our health and so distressing to millions of people throughout the world.

What IS the difference between fat and obesity? It is indeed very easy to become overweight in today's affluent and pleasure-seeking society where "eating out" has become such a part of enjoyment to so many. But, as we have all learned to our cost, it is far easier to put on those unwanted bulges than the uphill battle to lose them which can take weeks, months and, without help for many of us, never!

The human body has three separate kinds of fat which we must distinguish between, so as to understand what we are doing when we try to lose weight. First, there is structural fat, which is enveloped between the organs in the various parts of the body. It's a sort of protection, or packing material if you like, which keeps us comfortably together. This is necessary fat and should not be reduced under any circumstances.

The second kind of fat is the so called normal fat which is reserved for the energy purposes of the body. It is all over the body so that the system can draw freely when the nutritional intake is insufficient to meet the body's demands. This fat is a sort of bank deposit which is not immediately available but can be called upon any time the body needs extra reserves for excess muscular activity, extra energy requirements or to maintain our temperature. This fat is quite normal in its existence and cannot be called overweight or obesity.

The third type of fat is the trouble-maker and is completely abnormal. The problem is that this fat, collected up by all the extra unneeded calories which we stuff inside us, locks itself away in places like tummy, thighs, upper arms and hips and, however hard you diet, this abnormal fat tends to stay exactly where it is and exactly where you don't want it. Only as a last resort, and often not even then under normal diet conditions, will the body yield up this latent fat reserve.

However, I should point out here in fairness that it is possible to be statistically overweight – that is according to the much publicised weight tables – without actually being obese. Dr Pawan says that a national slimming survey of Britain shows that about half the population of Britain are overweight. Of these, 10% are over the weight ideal for their height. But obesity occurs in about a quarter of the total population and similar statistics are found in many Western countries.

There are some people who can gain or lose weight by their own will power over their calorie intake. These people are the lucky ones and can and do allow themselves at times to overeat, knowing they can control their weight easily themselves – which the obese person cannot.

Therefore, it all comes down to one fact – how and with what can we control that abnormal fat? After all, it's no good slimming ourselves silly if we are still going to end up with wobbly inner thighs and upper arms, bulging buttocks and hips and haggard faces!

Human Chorionic Gonadotropic Hormone
One of the most popular ways I have discovered of losing weight without tears is called HCG – a course of injections prescribed and administered by a doctor using a highly active substance called Human Chorionic Gonadotropic Hormone which has proved successful in many thousands of cases.

About 125 units of HCG is injected daily and the patient is allowed a daily dietary intake of 500 calories for a limited period of time – never more than forty consecutive days. The substance, HCG is highly active and produced in large quantities (up to one million international units daily) in the placenta of pregnant women, for the purpose of releasing the abnormal fatty deposit in the woman's body to make it available as energy for the growing foetus. It circulates in the mother's body and is excreted in the form of urine from which it is extracted. It is this hormone, in fact, which makes it possible for doctors to diagnose pregnancy from the commonly known urine test these days.

With a normal low calorie diet the first fat to go is usually the normal fatty tissue leaving the patient still with fat hips, thighs or abdomen – the areas which they originally set out to attack. With the aid of HCG doctors claim that it is these abnormal fatty areas that are disposed of first, leaving the normal fatty deposits alone in areas like the face and breasts from which one, particularly a woman, does not always want to lose weight!

Lady Cilento, the eminently respected Australian gynaecologist and nutrition expert and mother of actress Diane Cilento, has this to say: "It was found that this potent hormone was responsible for the strange phenomenon that pregnant women, although living on a meagre diet and even half starved, as they have been in famines and concentration camps, did not suffer the hardships of other women – hunger, fatigue, emaciation, sagging skin and weakness. They were able to mobilise their surplus fat to nourish their unborn babies. In abnormal times the baby had a constant supply of nourishment irrespective of the mother's own food fluctuations. Research has shown that when this same substance is introduced into the body of an ordinary person – irrespective of their age or sex – it mobilises their stored fat and uses that instead of the usual meals they would have eaten. Their bodies being constantly flooded with their own nourishment, they don't feel excessive craving for food. Nor does it drain away the normal subcutaneous fat that gives a rounded, youthful appearance to face and neck."

This being so, patients do not feel a constant craving for meals and yet they are left with their normal contours of bust, shoulders and breasts protected while the fatty supplies in areas of inner upper arms, thighs, buttocks and abdomen are used up and diminished.

I was interested to hear Lady Cilento's view that, "Only such minute quantities of HCG are needed to produce this decreased effect that in women there is no upset of normal periods, no interference with the efficacy of oral contraceptives (the Pill) and in men no feminising side effects."

The treatment is used extensively in the USA, London, France, many parts of Europe and Australia, and I can personally vouch for its effectiveness in large numbers of patients who I have seen through the course in perfect and vigorous health, ending up with super slim figures.

One girlfriend of mine had suffered from overweight for years and had tried every diet available, including Weightwatchers, with no effect. On HCG she became an attractive, slim young woman from a dumpy, miserable one in a period of just over four weeks.

Injections are usually given intramuscularly deep into the buttocks of 500 i.u. (international units) on alternate days, three times a week, or 125 i.u. per day for a maximum of forty days. There is usually an unrestricted diet for the first three days but from the fourth day onwards a strict 500 calorie regime. Patients can expect to lose three to five pounds a week.

Two meals a day can be eaten and may consist of the following: 4 ounces lean meat, veal, steak, beef, chicken breast, fish, sea food, prawns, crab, lobster, oysters, scallops weighed raw with all fat removed before grilling, boiling or steaming.

A normal serving of one low calorie vegetable or salad vegetable prepared without oil or butter. Use salt, pepper, vinegar, lemon juice as desired.

One unsweetend rusk or slice wholemeal bread, toast or biscuit is allowed. Also an apple, orange, pear, slice of paw paw, pineapple or grapefruit.

The quantity of fluid is unrestricted. As much water can be consumed as you wish, but you can only have one cup of tea, coffee (without sugar and with only one tablespoon of milk) in twenty-four hours. The juice of one lemon is allowed daily but a cup of Marmite, Vegemite, Promite, made with water, contains no calories at all! No other vitamins are allowed.

People wanting to lose excessive amounts of overweight fat can do a four to six week course, then return to a normal diet for a month or so before beginning another course.

One doctor, who has run one of the most successful slimming clinics in Australia using HCG and has personally supervised tens of thousands of patients in seventeen years, says, "I have not yet heard one case where there has been any negative effects from the use of HCG in any one person. There is no doubt in my mind that HCG in quantities we are discussing – that is one hundred and twenty five i.u. per day for a maximum of forty days – cannot have any harmful side effects."

In addition, of course, patients do have a daily consultation with their supervising doctors.

The treatment is used extensively in London by Phillip Lebon. In a latter to *The Lancet* in November 1966 he said: "I wish to stress that the use of HCG can lead to the loss of large amounts of weight while the patient is able to pursue an active working, social, and domestic life, and that my patients were able to contain within their treatment the burden of all the additional problems they were exposed to environmentally, and still do as well as, or even better than, patients admitted to hospital."

He submitted the following table showing the effect on weight of treatment with HCG:

Patient No.	Age	Dates of treatment	No. of dieting days	Starting & finishing weights (1 lb)	Weight loss	Remarks
1	12	21 April 1966	80	156/110	46	At school & holidays
2	62	1 July 1960	40	258/244	42	Professional singer and actor
3	45	15 July 1964 21 Nov. 1964 6 Dec. 1965	120	315/198	117	Tailor
4	37	11 Feb. 1966 10 June 1966	80	214/155	59	Secretary
5	40	7 Feb. 1966 13 July 1966	80	253/191	62	Company director
6	29	3 Nov. 1965 31 March 1966	60	242/183	59	Professional photographer
7	22	30 Dec. 1965	140	215/140	75	Housewife
8	21	16 April 1965 31 Aug. 1965	80	185/120	65	Secretary
9	34	15 June 1962 10 Oct. 1963	80	246/188	58	Company director
10	38	25 April 1963 11 April 1964	120	262/183	79	Restaurateur
11	49	12 Oct. 1960	80	169/126	43	Housewife diabetic

The treatment was first evolved by the well-known, late Dr A.T.W. Simeons, M.D., at his Salvator Mundi International Hospital in Monte Verde, Rome, who pioneered HCG nearly two decades ago, under whom many of the doctors now practising the treatment have studied. Certainly he was right when he quoted the old adage: "Inside every fat person there is a thin one crying to be let out!"

However, Dr Pawan who knew him, says that Simeons never claimed that HCG would work by itself. Pawan says, "It was always to be used with a 500 calorie diet and with the use of HCG people tend to stick to the diet more effectively. Everyone must lose weight if they eat less than they have been eating before."

The treatment has, of course, been strongly criticised by many doctors as there have been no clinical tests to show that it really works. I can only tell you that I have met many people personally on whom I have seen that it does work. The cost varies tremendously and I think is high. In London, for example, charges vary from around $300/£150 for three weeks.

Fat Mobilising Substance

One new idea which is being used in several parts of the world to good effect is FMS (Fat Mobilising Substance) which was first discovered by the nutritionist Dr Gaston Pawan, a consultant at the Middlesex Hospital Medical School, London. It is found in the urine of fasting or starving people – and it has been shown to have *exceptional* results in speeding up weight reduction in obese patients on a calorie controlled diet.

Dr Pawan's idea was to try and synthesise the material so that it can be used in sufficiently large quantities. However, medical research has shown that it is not particularly stable, and therefore it is difficult to use. In other words, its chemical make-up was likely to change during storage, over a period of several weeks. The many other doctors who had worked with FMS had experienced similar problems. To illustrate the difficulties involved in obtaining sufficient FMS: it requires 10 litres of urine from a fasting person to produce 15 milligrams of FMS which is equivalent to one injection, and it takes approximately 2 days of fasting for a person to produce 10 litres of urine.

A doctor who suggested obtaining FMS from the people of starving countries, such as Bangladesh, by setting up clinics to collect urine as a source of income, was medically and publicly shot down in flames for his "outrageous" idea. However, the fact remains that FMS has been shown to mobilise fat to speed its breakdown under strict diet conditions, and research into treatment continues. It is being used on slimming patients in Hungary and at a number of clinics in the United States.

Bio feedback Training
I think a far more realistic approach to our dietary and nutrition problems is along psychological lines, to treat the cause and not the symptoms and the cause of overeating is almost always psychological.

Thomas Beck, who has been working as an obesity consultant for years, says he believes he has found an answer. It is Bio feedback Training – the application of learning to control our own brain wave activity by getting a feed-back when the brain is functioning in an alpha state, that is the sign of relaxation and creativity. Once we learn how to relax at will and, as a result, naturally, we would eliminate all compulsive eating habits.

After all, you eat compulsively when you have some sort of tensions, anxieties, stress which drives you to food as a compensation for other frustrations in life. If you could relax at will this would be eliminated. So, says Tom Beck, the idea is to teach some relaxation techniques that they can easily master. "Most people have no idea how to relax. The word relax is very badly understood. If you ask somebody to relax they usually tense up. If I ask you to fly an areoplane you couldn't do it because you've never had the experience before. Therefore, you have to experience relaxation before you can do it.

"To this end, we have a new method called autogenic training which is a derivation of auto-hypnosis and we are using a completely new modality which has never been used in psychology before called Relative Analgesia. It is used in dentistry for the purpose of not killing pain or not blocking the passage of pain through the nervous system but to raise the threshold of pain reception, thereby causing us not to be aware of pain. It's a combination of an old anaesthetic called nitrousoxide, otherwise known as laughing gas, which was used in anaesthetics all round the world. Only in the last few years in the U.S. have they started to use nitrous-oxide in combination with oxygen for the so-called relative analgesia, mostly in dentistry and now even in obstetrics during childbirth, where the oxygen content of the mixture is controlled by the equipment to such an extent that it cannot induce total analgesia. It can only induce a state of mind where the perception of pain is not as intensive as it was before. You are completely awake and aware of happenings around you and it produces a pleasant 'high' as when taking alcohol or marihuana. You are just floating, pleasantly on cloud nine without being aware or caring about the pain induced. We are not using it for reasons of pain but to teach people to relax.

"Once they are consciously aware of a relaxation state, we give them suggestions during that time because the sub-conscious is wide open to suggestion. We can suggest they regress food or habits during the treatment period, like being able to resist a chocolate cake or ice cream or whatever . . . We use this period to give them suggestions of how to cope with this problem in the future. The idea is unique in the world.

"Before we begin treatment of course, we have to know the eating history and problems. We don't talk about a diet, for a start. We speak of food management or a nutritional management plan. We ask people to give us an exact diary of what they are eating in one week; how much they are eating, when they are eating it, where they are eating it and who with, under what circumstances and conditions. Taking this diary we then develop a plan for nutrition that is within their normal eating habits, but won't change their day-to-day pattern of life and they don't have to cook something separate. They continue to eat basically the same things with the exception of primarily all carbohydrates. You can eliminate all carbohydrates, then reintroduce them gradually over the weeks, each week giving them a little bit more until such time as the total weight is lost. After that we try to establish each individual's optimum carbohydrate level which would maintain the sole weight achieved.

"On the psychological side, we try to establish what caused their abnormal eating habits, whether it goes back to their childhood, or even babyhood, or whether they were gradually acquired due to frustrations, tensions, stresses, etc., or due to external influences such as new family habits of husband or wife, social economical influences such as not being able to afford nutritionally good food but having to stick to starch-rich diets like pastas, which are very common in the Italian communities, rice in Chinese communities, or bread in the middle European groups with potatoes, etc. Once the causes are established, then the practitioner can proceed to give the patients something tangible, an impulse for achieving results under relaxation on a psychological level."

Calories
Most of us are sufficiently aware to know that too many calories mean too much fat and that we all have our ideal calorie intake per day depending on our height and ideal average weight. The older we get, generally speaking, the less calories per day we require.

However, whatever our diet, most of us need to cheat a little with an in-between snack. Here are a few low calorie nibbles that could help to see you through a difficult day. After all, you can always deduct the extra total from dinner or supper so that you keep your daily quota intact.

Food	Calories
1 apple	80
1 banana	85
1 raw carrot	25
cup fresh cherries	80
1 oz Swiss cheese	95
1 oz Camembert cheese	85
1 oz raisins	60
1 peach	35
¼ honeydew melon	65
1 orange	60

1 slice Ryvita (no butter)	26
half cup Yoghurt with honey	100

Body Servicing Diet

This diet is for weight control, beauty, health, vigour and longevity. It recommends you to take one strong multi-vitamin (Gevral or Phamaton) per day and permits tea or decaffeinated coffee in limited quantities with skimmed milk, sweetener or honey. It excludes all oil, fat, cream, sugar, flour or added salt. You may substitute one meal for another provided you eat the liver as prescribed and you may eat the 3 meals given in each day's menu, in any order you like.

DAY 1

Breakfast

One multi-vitamin tablet. Fresh orange juice. One slice of wholewheat bread and peanut butter. One cup of coffee or tea with skimmed milk and sweetener.

Lunch

4 ounce tin of sardines (drain off oil). Beetroot and lettuce salad (wine vinegar dressing). One cup of tea or coffee or one glass of skimmed milk.

Dinner

One glass of vegetable or tomato juice. Grilled lean steak with boiled cauliflower. One cup of tea or coffee.

DAY TWO

Breakfast

One multi-vitamin tablet. One poached or boiled egg. One slice of wholewheat bread, toasted. One cup of tea or coffee.

Lunch

Half a cold chicken. Raw salad including celery and radishes. One sliced orange. One cup of tea or coffee.

Dinner

One ounce unsalted nuts. Large portion of grilled cod, grilled mushrooms and a small tin of asparagus. One cup of tea or coffee.

DAY THREE
Breakfast
One multi-vitamin tablet. One glass of skimmed milk.
Lunch
One ounce of unsalted nuts. One glass of V.8 (mixed vegetable) juice. Prawns and mixed salad. One cup of tea or coffee.
Dinner
One cup of beetroot soup. Grilled liver, two onions cooked in the oven and spinach. Two slices of pineapple. One cup of tea or coffee.

DAY FOUR
Breakfast
One multi-vitamin tablet. One glass fresh grapefruit juice. One slice of wholewheat bread, toasted, and honey. One cup of tea or coffee.
Lunch
Two slices of cold roasted meat, raw cabbage, celery, radishes and onion salad. Fresh fruit salad. One cup of tea or coffee.
Dinner
One ounce unsalted nuts. Large portion of salmon, with peas and soya beans.

DAY FIVE
Breakfast
One multi-vitamin tablet. Six halves of stewed apricots (without sugar). One cup of tea or coffee.
Lunch
Tomato juice. Two lean grilled lamb chops. Lentils and green salad. One cup of tea or coffee.
Dinner
One cup of consommé. Large portion of grilled fish with lemon. Spinach or cauliflower. One fresh citrus fruit. One cup of tea or coffee.

DAY SIX
Breakfast
One multi-vitamin tablet. One glass of prune juice. One slice of wholewheat bread and soya spread. One cup of tea or coffee.
Lunch
One ounce unsalted nuts. Half a grilled chicken. Grilled mushrooms and peas. Half fresh grapefruit. One cup of tea or coffee.
Dinner
Seafood cocktail with wine vinegar. One veal chop. Boiled cabbage. Small bunch of fresh grapes. One cup of tea or coffee.

DAY SEVEN
Breakfast
One multi-vitamin tablet. One glass of fresh orange juice. One cup of tea or coffee.
Lunch
Large portion of roast beef or lamb with peas, cabbage, and carrots. Fresh fruit salad. One cup of tea or coffee.
Dinner
Shell fish or fish of your choice with mixed salad. One cup of tea or coffee.

Peanut butter, soya spread, lentils, wholewheat bread, etc. are available from any health food shop.

Protein Diet
One of the most effective and fast-working diets of all I have found is the all protein diet. You must stick rigidly to the rules and allow not one scrap of carbohydrate to pass your lips – otherwise all is ruined. The trouble is most of us imagine that it is expensive, as the only real protein we can think of on an everday basis is either steak or chicken. However, there are many other tasty forms of protein containing far less calories than, say, a 3 oz sirloin steak which has 330 calories supplying 20 grams of protein. What you should be aiming for is 1 gram of protein per day for every two pounds you weigh – therefore if you are an average of 130 pounds you should aim to take 65 grams of protein per day.

But the protein diet certainly rips off the overweight pounds. Here are some good protein buys that will make up some varied low calorie meals. As you will see, a protein diet need NOT be a bore, too, which puts most of us off trying it in the first place.

Weight (ozs)	Food	Protein content in grams	Calories
3	Canned salmon	17	120
2.4	Round steak (lean only, broiled)	21	130
3	Canned crabmeat	15	85
4	Uncreamed cottage cheese	17	85
3	Broiled chicken	20	115
2.6	Lean lamb chop (without fat)	21	140
4	Bean sprouts (raw)	3	23
1	Natural Swiss cheese	8	105
2	Fried liver	15	130
3	Baked fish (not in oil)	22	135
3	Canned shrimps	21	100
4	Natural oysters	10	80
3	Corned beef	22	185
3	Canned sardines (no oil allowed)	20	175

The important thing is that all of us should take a new look at ourselves and our eating habits in relation to our health. There is no doubt through all my researches that nutrition – although doctors and scientists are only just touching the tip of the iceberg – holds the key to the majority of the health problems that beset the world today. The awareness of many families in planning the daily diet, the popularity of health food shops, the interest in organically grown foods are all terrific steps forward.

None of us can afford to ignore the relationship between our food, our health and our chances of longer life. Keeping ourselves fit and slim is only step one on the long road to longevity and a healthier, more active old age.

I should just like to add a cautionary note: please be sure to check with your doctor before embarking on any attempt to cure overweight or obesity by dieting

CHAPTER TWENTY-THREE

A Death Hormone: Tripping The Time Clock

"There's no way of escaping it"

Dr W. Donner Denckla
Roche Institute of Molecular Biology,
New Jersey, U.S.A.

If we are seriously intrigued by the questions of eternal youth and the possibilities of increased longevity, the inevitable question for all of us to ask is – what next? Where can science possibly take us in the next few decades? The answer, according to at least one eminent biochemist, is a chance that we could live forever – or at least for centuries so that we become our own walking history book. He says he has found a previously hitherto untraced compound secreted by the pituitary gland, at the base of the brain, called a Decreasing Oxygen Consumption Hormone (DECO). If he can isolate it, remove it, re-programme it and return it to the pituitary (which he claims is only a matter of a few years' work), man could technically be immortalised. He says: "The body is perfectly capable of living for centuries."

In addition, the biochemist claims that he has already found the elusive secret of eternal life – that in laboratory experiments with rats he has, in fact *reversed* the ageing process from the equivalent of sixty years to twenty! Of course, as we know, most gerontologists have long been of the opinion that we should be able to live naturally to at least around one hundred and twenty years of age. But Dr W. Donner Denckla, the brilliant chief biochemist with the Roche Drug Company Institute of Molecular Biology in Nutley, New Jersey, U.S.A., goes one giant step further. Denckla, whether his theories are finally accepted or not, is indeed a brilliant scientist.

He began his experiments in late 1969. He is a tall, rangy-looking American, who talks fast and intensely to put over his ideas, anxious you should follow his thinking every step of the incredible way through the whole history of evolution from birth to death.

Denckla made his discoveries while working specifically in finding treatments for the problems of ageing as part of his work at the Roche Laboratories. His idea of eternal life does indeed today sound like so much science fiction. But is it? Denckla is no crazy scientist. He is a man with an undoubtedly brilliant and imaginative brain, highly regarded by colleagues all over the world. Certainly what he has to say is worth our consideration. If Denckla's process theories can be proven beyond any shadow of doubt – and he says they can – then the very basis of our civilisation as we know it will have been turned upside down.

The far reaching questions for mankind are so mind-boggling that they are almost without answer. Can you imagine, for example, living for seven hundred years or more? Can you envisage being on earth at the same time as all the rest of your own family tree? Can you imagine spreading out a career, a number of careers, your store of educational knowledge over generations? Worse, can you imagine facing up to the stresses and troubles of not one lifetime as we know it now but hundreds of years of similar, never ending problems? Can you even guess at the wealth, the possessions, the fortunes, the homes some people would amass? The problems of the population explosion, ecology, food, water, the sociological upheavals in a world already over-populated and over-polluted. Finally, what would be the ultimate decisions of world government on which of the breed would be allowed to live and reproduce and which of us would have, for the survival of the race, to be eliminated?

These problems Denckla can foresee but as he told me: "I am a scientist. I just make the discoveries. The problems, I am afraid, will have to be faced by higher authorities than I."

As, indeed, the problems of the atom bomb, the H bomb and nuclear arms in today's world have been the ultimate responsibility not of the scientists but of our world leaders. The whole idea, of course, is beyond the immediate comprehension of you and I, but what of the theory behind it all? I have spent many an hour seated before a blackboard in the laboratory at the Denckla's family home in New Jersey as he pounded out his ideas and conclusions in careful detail.

As I outlined earlier in discussing his theories in relation to our chances of living to the 22nd century, Dr Denckla is one of many scientists working on the theory that ageing and death is caused by the tripping of a time clock. They believe that there is a time clock somewhere within the human brain which, however healthy we are, triggers off and ensures we die at around our allotted time. As Denckla says, death has to be a natural part of evolution in exactly the same way as is birth. What the boffins have been after, particularly the Russians, is to find the time clock and discover a way of re-programming it to allow us to control our own key to survival. Chebotarev in Kiev is rumoured to have claimed he has done it, but no certain evidence from the Russians has been forthcoming.

I was the first writer that Denckla had talked to about his astounding discoveries, based on the new hormone (DECO). The general theory behind the Time Clock of Ageing is that at a certain time it emits an enzyme or hormone which completely blankets all the other bodily systems, most importantly of all the DNA or nucleus of the cell, and cancels them out, like a computer of the brain that says, "Time is up."

Denckla began by looking at the main reasons for death in mammals. It seems strange, he said, that out of the hundreds of ways we can die of disease, all finally break down to three main reasons: lack of blood; infections; neoplasm.

These add up to the failure of the immunological system. This breaks down for two main reasons: lack of blood and immunology. So, says Denckla, it would seem that if we can cure both of these things we should be able to live for all time. Yet even since the seventeenth century doctors have been trying to find a solution to curing death – without success.

However, here he goes back to the theory of evolution. "I am of the opinion," he says, "that death is completely, utterly and absolutely purposeful. Evolution will not work without death. In higher animals death has to occur. Death is a mechanism of cleaning out the brush and allowing new growth to come up through the dead wood. A different growth – that's the important thing. Evolution requires different growth. From the point of view of the individual, death is tragedy and birth is joyous. But from the point of view of the species it is just as necessary to kill off as to give birth. What really matters in time is the species and there's no damn room unless you kill off the original species. You have to develop a heavy fur coat to provide for winter and you're going to have to kill off all the animals with thin coats. If you can imagine looking into a time tunnel which goes deep back maybe a billion years – and this is a tunnel of life – the only important factor, and this is a truism everybody learns in the first year of biology, is you are a linear descendant of the first living organism, by definition. Uninterrupted your proto-plasm is essentially a living descendant of the first swiggly little bacteria and it won't spring from some mountain peak. Therefore animals must be able to adapt to the changes in environment.

"You must allow new forms of life to spring forth in the presence of new environmental changes. This is where death becomes a completely essential thing."

In higher animals death has to occur. Therefore a time clock has been built into each and every one of us to ensure that we do die. What causes the clock to work? There has to be something which can act between the clock and the body. Says Denckla: "I came to the conclusion that it must be a hormone."

Now, what we are trying to say is that if you accept the fact that the biological clock runs puberty, gestation and growth and the heart rate and metabolic rate – whatever we choose – then it must also run the life span. But an ordinary clock can do no more than tell the time. This clock of the brain must have some sort of trigger. Therefore we must have a brain and clock producing some hormones on schedule which likewise produce an effect which is either developmental or timed.

How do we know hormones are involved? Well, for example – "if I take out your pituitary, you will not be able to reproduce. If I take out your ovaries, you will not be able to reproduce. If I take out your thyroid, you will not be able to reproduce. If I take them out in puberty you won't go through puberty. If I cut a certain section in your heart, your heart will stop. The metabolic rate is controlled by the thyroid. The arm of the clock controls all these events. And if the same clock controls them then presumably the same class of effectors is in turn bringing about the demise of the system. So reasoning that we can go back and we can say that the X factor which causes the failure of our two systems, the cardio-vascular and the immune, is probably the hormones, so, that which stands between the clock and our death is also probably a hormone."

For that reason Dr Denckla started his search for the new and previously unspotted all powerful hormone. He was almost certain that he was right, that there was such a hormone and that he would find it.

His aim was to find the X factor and block it.

And it had to be a major hormone, otherwise it wouldn't have the strength and power to kill. It had to be a hormone involved directly or indirectly with normal development. Now there are two major hormones. The Thyroid hormone, called Thyroxine and its right hand maiden Thioritothyronene – T3 and T4. Science does not know which one is the leading one and both are active biologically. Nothing normal happens in the body's development unless these two hormones are also normal. Denckla backtracked to investigations that had been made by earlier scientists seventy years ago and then ignored, and found that the key seemed to be in the oxygen consumption of these two hormones compared with every other hormone in the body.

Dr Denckla said that he found that the DECO was quite capable of putting out a blanket that could cloak every life supporting system in the body, including the vital source of life itself, the DNA or very nucleus of the cells. "If you take the pituitary gland out the mantle disappears," he says. Denckla only finalised this part of his studies, involving long hours of mathematical analysis, in the early part of 1976. "It was a puzzle eluding scientists for years," he said "I am not saying that it is the decreasing oxygen consumption hormone that kills you, but that it does cause the decrease in the systems which are the key for survival."

The next step, he says, is removing the hormone from the pituitary and re-programming it. Theoretically, he knows exactly how to do it all. "All I need is enough finance and man hours in the form of scientific help to do it. It would take us less than five years."

Five years to find the key to eternal life! Very many scientists will be waiting to do battle with Dr Denckla on his theory. Let us stand on the sidelines and just watch with interest.

CHAPTER TWENTY-FOUR

Fiji – Health And Beauty All Under One Blue Sky!

"Stimulate the Phagocytes – Drugs are a Delusion."

George Bernard Shaw

The girl sitting opposite me that morning at breakfast was beautiful. There was no other word for her. Blonde, blue eyed, she had that clear transparent sort of skin, the colour of warm honey, over which the beauty advertisers spend thousands annually in the hope of helping the rest of us to achieve it. Yet her hands were shaking as she stirred cream into her coffee.

She knew my eyes were on her. "Yes," she admitted, as if reading my unspoken questions, "I *am* worried. In fact, if you really want to know, I am scared stiff."

Two hours later, I knew, Margot, a rich broker's wife from Australia was due to undergo her first ever course of cell therapy. She was only twenty-eight! Only a few months earlier I'd have been surprised and shocked, too. Why should a girl so young and attractive be even worrying about her looks-never mind taking such lengths to preserve them?

However, by the time we met I was already well aware that there is today a whole new breed of Beautiful People, growing in every class and facet of society, who not only realise the increasing importance and potential of rejuvenation methods in modern day medicine but are also determined to take advantage of them. They are the people of all ages who are eager to do all they can to stay looking young and beautiful and remain healthy for as many years as nature can be prevailed upon to allow.

I have already emphasised that not one doctor but many today believe a healthy 120 years old to be more of a natural life span than the short 70 or 80 we are currently led to expect, if we are lucky. Yet, still I can see the elderly among my own acquaintances preparing to opt out around then, as if they have had the most that can be expected and feel themselves fairly privileged not to have been struck down like their more unfortunate colleagues who died from coronaries and the like in their forties!

What nonsense it is to be so utterly brain-washed by the past and our own history books. Isn't every other facet of our life around us changing our views on everything we thought sacrosanct from money to morals? And Margot was just typical of the new breed of today's Beautiful People who want to remain the beautiful, talented and successful of tomorrow, too. And why not?

She was among the first of hundreds of patients already flying into Fiji to visit what is being planned as the world's finest rejuvenation clinic – a unique US$4,000,000 health hotel and hospital which will include – under one roof – all the leading treatments available from scientists dedicating their lives to the study of prolonged youth and longevity, all round the globe.

It is, of course, planned as a super blueprint for the youth clinics of the future. It is a twenty-first century dream centre, a science fiction, style press-button health and beauty farm-plus, where you can holiday and get a top-to-toe body refit and fuel change at one and the same time. It will be the sort of place where the busy executive, who would ideally like to spend his precious annual holidays at a health farm but also wants to have his cake and eat it by fishing, riding and lazing through a tropical island's holiday pleasures, can truly find the best of both worlds.

It is an idea that is catching on and no wonder – with holidaymakers from Japan, the South East Asia region, South Pacific, Australia, New Zealand and America. Which is why I was there on the spot in one of the world's most romantic and idyllic holiday resorts, Pacific Harbour on the Coral Coast of the Fijian Islands. Here at this crossroads of world holiday travel, there are plans to build a health hotel that overlooks the frothing, spectacular coastal seascapes on the one hand and lies close by one of the world's finest international golf courses which spreads with manicured precision panoramically across the valley like a green velvet carpet, the tranquility only occasionally broken by the movement of one of those American-style electric caddy carts buzzing across the greens.

What exactly is a health hotel? I was as curious as everyone else when I first arrived at Nadi International airport to find out what the boffins had in mind. I transferred, after a good night's sleep, to a tiny Fijian Airways internal flight to wing my way right across the heart of the densely jungled and sugar cane country, a cloud-topped Shangri-La which is the interior of mainland Fiji towards the far coast and the capital Suva. There on a tiny airstrip, 36 miles from Suva by road, I discovered the gem that is Pacific Harbour, a spot I wish I could keep to myself for its peace and beauty, but which is destined to become world famous in the rejuvenation field.

Most people, who want to operate at peak efficiency in health today, are the very people who lack one vital commodity in their lives – time. They haven't the time to fly hither and thither searching for treatments for their looks, their figures, their weight control, their wrinkles, their sex lives or their neuroses. They might like to visit a cosmetic surgeon and have their eyes de-bagged; or a super-slick clinic in South America which gives cell therapy and deep sea compression treatments – most effectively, they say – combined. They'd probably love to try cell therapy, or B-15 or a dozen different treatments. But who has the time to fly around taking a tuck up here or removing a wrinkle there, and get that much needed vital rest only an annual holiday in the sun can provide?

At Pacific Harbour the idea is that we have all of this rolled into one beautiful package. And for the visitor thirsting after youth and health there could not be a more idyllic spot on earth. It will be tailored to provide a service for anyone from the working man to the top executive, who can save up the price of an all in one package holiday - that is if you don't want all the extras like plastic surgery thrown in.

Pacific Habour was born originally out of a dream. Once a mango swamp on the "wrong side" of the island, as the old British

Colonialists would have had it in their day in Fiji, it has been built into the magnificent resort it is today thanks to the persistence and vision of one man. A New Zealander, Pat Samuels, first fell in love with Fiji when he was flying over the Pacific during the last war. He saw a dazzling strip of white sand between the azure of the coral reef and the dark green of the Fijian inland mountain peaks. That, he told himself, was one of the most beautiful natural seascapes he had ever seen. He went on to Canada to end up after the war as head of one of the world's largest international car firms. But he never forgot his Fiji and frequently returned to holiday there and visit the spot which, he said, could be made into the Pacific's finest resort, with beaches to rival, or even surpass, Rio's Copocabana, Sydney's Bondi and Bangladesh's still undeveloped Cox's Bazaar.

His suggestion, of course, was received with nothing but scorn from friends. After all, Pacific Harbour was then little more than a mango swamp. But Samuels was not to be put off. Moving among his many friends in high business circles, he pushed, weedled and bullied until by the early 1960's he persuaded two Canadian business associates to join him. They formed a company to purchase a small sixteen acre site. It included an old wooden hotel built there years earlier as part of the sets for the famous Burt Lancaster epic, *His Majesty O'Keefe.*

Foreigners, of course, cannot normally buy large tracts of land in Fiji which is, on the whole, Crown Property. But mango swamps? Well, at that time they were up for grabs. And Pat Samuels was making a giant snatch to make his long time dream come true. By 1969 the men realised that if their plan was to become reality it must be on a much larger scale, and they accumulated some 7400 acres around their original small plot and re-named the area Pacific Harbour. Then planning began in earnest. Top experts on everything from construction to waterways, electric power, engineering and ecology – to preserve or replace the natural beauty of the place after building – were brought in from all over the world. One of them was Robert Trent-Jones, the American golf course designer, who was responsible for the magnificent seventy-two par eighteen-hole championship course that exists there today.

The whole area is a tropical paradise. Already well over one hundred private villas, most of them with swimming pools, traditional Tapa decor and cool arched roofs, have been developed and sold privately. There is a magnificent hotel, the Beachcomber, on the site of the old Burt Lancaster original – now one of the most luxurious in the Pacific region. There are tarmac roads, a new shopping centre with old colonnaded colonial-style stores and local crafts centres, and even a new marina from where the watersport-loving holidaymaker can go cruising, reef fishing or big game hunting for marlin and shark which abound in these waters. The golf course, with fine swimming pool and clubhouse of its own, is already attracting top class golfers from the world international circuits.

When Fijian health authorities first heard the suggestion of the arrival of a Health Hotel and Clinic, and eventually a combined hospital at Pacific Harbour, they were decidedly dubious and even suspicious. The easy-going islanders with their healthy carefree life-style don't, after all, worry too much about stress, the rat-race and all the everyday problems of the rough and tumble of the rest of the outside world. They didn't want to get involved in what advisers over in Australia's Health Authorities regarded as "fringe" medicine. As I have said, the Australians cling closely to medical beliefs and regulations of their equally cagey American counterparts.

But slowly, step by step, in the way that Pat Samuels had achieved the initial plan in creating Pacific Harbour at all, the planners unfolded the medical evidence to show that Fiji could indeed have a splendid world first with a health hotel. It would attract many more thousands of tourists to one of the most talked about combined health and holiday spots in the world, in addition to providing more jobs for Fijians. So, in early 1977, the first moves were made in the Parliament towards laying the foundations of Bula-Bula – the Fijian word for welcome, by which the centre is already known to locals.

All under one blue sky, the centre is already offering visitors some of the best treatments from the world youth supermarket in one holiday health luxury package. Guests, at present, who are combining holidays with treatment, stay at the Beachcomber

Hotel or in privately rented villas. But when the complex is completed, during the next two years, accommodation will be the ultimate in luxury. There will be split-level apartments, each with their own private balconies and superb views over the coastline. There will be fabulous international cuisine and special gourmet diets for those intent on losing weight. Holidaymakers will be able to come to the hotel purely for a holiday if they wish, and they won't have to take any cure other than the fresh air and sunshine or the many pleasures laid on such as riding, snorkelling, swimming, fishing, picnicking, pedal-carring, sailing, whether in a Fijian out-rigger or a luxury launch, or just wining, dining and sunning. The health and revitalisation facilities, use of saunas, gymnasiums and massage treatments will also be available to guests at other villas and hotels at the same fees as to the health hotel visitors.

What treatments will the Beautiful People find there? The list makes me gasp. The hotel has drawn on so many international experts in youth treatments. For a start everyone will get a full medical check-up and for the tired out executive there will be a complete top to toe overhaul. Treatments will eventually include, cell therapy, RNA and DNA therapy, B.15, Aslan or KH3 therapy, serum therapy, thalasso (sea water) therapy, massage, mud therapies for Europe, bio feedback and relaxation techniques. Weight control will be a big programme, with HCG for people who want to do it seriously under medical surveillance, as well as diet plans for the fitness addict who simply wants to shed a few evasive pounds. There will be treatments available, too, for those suffering from anxiety and stress, also help with sexual problems.

Eventually it is planned to have a top class plastic surgery section adjoining the hotel. This will also house a special HBO Hyperbaric Unit which will be available for providing emergency help from anywhere in Fiji.

The idea of putting all these treatments under one roof is certain to be only one of many springing up during the next decade. Plans already include copies of the health hotel and clinic in the Black Sea area, the Middle East and North Africa. Guests are travelling from as far afield as Japan, the Phillipines, Far East, Taiwan, Australia, New Zealand and the United States.

The point that pleases me about the idea is that it is not just for rich men but for anyone who can afford a modest holiday in the sun.

CHAPTER TWENTY-FIVE

The Final Diagnosis

Summing it all up, where does it lead us - this mystical, magical road to Shangri-La? I said, right at the outset, that I am personally convinced that there *is* a modern day fountain of youth – and I still hold firmly to that belief.

However, for the novice and the unwary it is a confusing road to travel, with its many claims and counter claims; the tempting little offbeat lanes and byeways that can lead all to easily, expensively and disappointingly to nowhere at all . . . But who shall we trust? What choices can we or dare we make to give ourselves the best possible individual chance of retaining our youth – assuming we have made the decision to step into the world of alternative medicine?

I have tried, with painstaking care, throughout my journey to analyse and evaluate all I have seen and heard. To separate fact from so much that is fake and fantasy. To tell you how and why and where so many other people are getting what they believe is a new lease on life, to discuss the offbeat as well as the mainstream thinking in rejuvenation, based on serious research.

I strongly believe that many of these still controversial, new ways of beating old age will become regarded as the medical norm of the 1980's and 90's. Of this there can be no doubt. But as yet there are no short cuts. There is no single miraculous wonder cure – no Goddess of Youth sitting beckoning, holding the ultimate solution – bottled youth in a pill or pot. So let's look at what we do have and try to pinpoint several indisputable conclusions.

Since embarking on my research project, I have focussed closely on the signs, the ravages, the cruelties and pain, as well as many of the triumphs of people in coping with age.

My travels across the world, among thousands of people of all social backgrounds and cultures, have only served to underline that there are, without doubt, many new and scientific ways at our disposal to help us stay young and enjoy the fitness, health and vitality of youth right through our later years – if we will take them. There are now tens of thousands of people – many more than you could ever guess – who are already seeking out and benefitting from these new methods. People everywhere are sharing an increasing burning curiosity to know more about their chances of staying young.

The new ball game for those in the know is to stay younger longer – leaving your school friends behind. The secret is to make sure that it is not the other way around. And it is, as I have tried to prove to you, something you can talk about without being regarded as a vain freak.

As we approach the 21st century, we no longer need to accept as a matter of course that we have to buckle down to the miserable shackles of old age, aches, pains, sickness and infirmity. And why should we? In the next century I believe that youth therapies in general, rejuvenation methods and treatments for many of the hitherto hopeless diseases of ageing, including heart and arthritic conditions, will be developed and indeed become a part of ordinary conventional every day medicine. Asking the doctor for help in staying young won't mean you'll be laughed out of the waiting room. It will be as ordinary as asking for a contraceptive pill or a slimming aid to help reduce your weight.

Some of these new developments could perhaps be here much sooner than we think, well before the year 2000. Already in the last decade, we can see the great strides forward that have been made toward world-wide recognition of many of the controversial rejuvenation treatments I have mentioned. Recall, for example, that many more sympathetic conventional G.P.'s will already obtain Gerovital, KH3, B-15 and even cell therapy jabs privately for patients on prescription, although they claim officially to regard them as so much psychological rubbish.

Meanwhile, out of all the treatments I have mentioned, has one more merit than another? All I can say is I have written about the leading treatments in explicit detail so that individual seekers after youth and health can make up their minds for themselves. After all, much depends on your age and what you are hoping to achieve from rejuvenation. Whether you are like the beautiful, blonde girl I met in Fiji who, at the age of twenty-eight, was investing in cell therapy. She is one of a whole new breed of young and beautiful people who want to stay as they are for as long as they can, thanks to alternative medicine. Many others, less concerned about their looks, may be more anxious to improve their sex drive, their memory retention or treat any number of the medical problems of ageing. The choice of treatment, therefore, must be dictated entirely by personal circumstances and medical factors.

I have written of my own personal experiences of cell therapy. I went into it with the complete scepticism of the journalist. I have to admit, however, that I felt younger, better and generally healthier for many months after it and I shall try it again. However, there are many thousands of others who swear by their own special brand of youth treatment, bearing in mind that not all of us can afford to fly off on a two week package holiday to have our youth jabs in the sun. Others – many millions – rely on daily pills bought over the chemist's counter as their own way of keeping age at bay with apparently excellent results.

Ideally, of course, one should consult one's own doctor about any proposed treatment. But in this field of alternative medicine many of them have no more – and sometimes less – knowledge on the subject than you yourself. Even if your doctor privately agrees with your decision to have a course of youth therapy, he is unlikely to approve it officially. And ethically one can appreciate his position. Fortunately, the majority of youth clinics are run by medically qualified doctors and if you are worried, you can check this for yourself before embarking.

Curiously, I have found several common denominators running through all the most successful youth treatments – too obvious to ignore. There is no question that nutrition, a carefully balanced diet and weight control are of vital importance in everything connected with health, youth and a successful sex life. Oxygen, too, obviously plays a leading role in the whole rejuvenation pattern, although exactly how has not yet been defined by scientists. Finally, the cells themselves, the condition and treatment of the millions upon millions of tiny cells of which each bodily organ and bodily system is made up, are another vital key to how young we look and feel.

I will not attempt to go into an in-depth analytical discussion of a subject too complex for even our most eminent scientists to understand. I am just throwing out, purely as observations, some of the salient factors on which scientists are even now working to find the link. You will recall that the most long-lived races – the Hunzacuts, the Caucasians and Ecuadorians – all live in high, mountainous regions, in which they breathe rarified oxygen; their oxygen consumption is increased by walking up and down hilly terrain. Hyperbaric treatment, too, owes its success to the bombardment of the system with pure oxygen under pressure in simulated deep sea dives. B-15 also is shown to owe its rejuvenation effects to instant oxygenation of the cells, increasing the supply of oxygen to every part of the body. But it is in the regeneration and stimulation of the cells of the body that most scientists believe lies the ultimate key.

Most of the more successful rejuvenation treatments are in some way involved with regeneration of the cell or the RNA. and DNA. at the very source of nucleus of the cell itself. It is the regeneration of imperfect cells damaged by infection, disease, strain, alcohol, nicotine and so on, as well as the many stresses of life, that causes the body slowly to degenerate and age. Therefore it doesn't need a scientific mind to see that any treatment involving replacement of perfect cells would seem to hold at least a part of the answer.

Fortunately for all of us, serious research is expanding all the time by scientists delving for the ultimate answer. Their dream, and ours, I suppose if we are honest, is to find the super pill or legendary elixir which is going to turn back the clock, wipe away the signs of ageing and give us back our youth. There is, as yet, no way we can achieve this instant transformation of our dreams, the secret for which men and women have searched for centuries. Perhaps, thankfully I say, there never will be.

To look young and youthful, to retain the supple skin and muscle tone of our 20's and 30's, to age gracefully and gradually is an aim for which it is worth striving. Many of these things are now possible and scientists are working closer all the time to the ultimate goal of probing the mechanism that causes ageing. But to be able to reverse totally the ageing process, to achieve our youth all over again as casually as we might change our hair style, or flick over the page of a book, I believe would be a terrifying prospect.

There are already strong claims, as I have reported, from responsible researchers that experiments have been completed to reverse successfully the ageing process in animals. That it should be possible in humans is conceivably, therefore, only a matter of time. Again, there are hints that it is already accomplished.

But is it something we truly want – the ultimate secret of youth? Controlled, it would indeed be a valuable weapon – a means of easing our way slowly through our middle and later years with the vigour and health of our youth.

Imagine how fantastic it would be at 90 to have the vitality of a 19-year-old! At 50 to have the smooth attractive skin of when we were 30. But the possibility of man being able to reverse his age at will into a second or third childhood – a Peter Pan society in which we could plunge backwards into our own children's generation or even our grandchildrens' – poses a range of horrors in emotional, social and genetic terms hitherto unthought of outside the realms of science fiction. It is equivalent to the similar promise – I say threat – by some scientists that before long they may know how to keep us alive for several hundreds of year. No. It is better to accept the scientists' view that age is a simple fact of all-known life – as autumn follows the spring.

But there is nothing against today's viewpoint that, with the help of science, we may enjoy a much longer spring before we begin to lose that youthful bloom. The ultimate success of science is surely to give us a chance to live longer – better. And, believe me, those chances in the coming decades are getting better all the time.

The question is whether you have the courage to reach out and grab them. Who really in their hearts wants to exchange youth for wisdom if that wisdom must be accompanied by the cracks, ugliness and ravages of the years? Certainly not me, if there's a single potion on the shelf, a single safe jab or wonder cure round the corner to ease the growing. That's why so many of us today are thirsting for knowledge of the ways we can make it happen. The knowledge of how to stay young – by any means possible.

Personally, I feel if I have given a few people just a little hope of coping better with the advances of age and their own enjoyment of life – then my travels have been worth while.